Practical Immunopathology of the Skin

CURRENT CLINICAL PATHOLOGY

IVAN DAMJANOV, MD
SERIES EDITOR

Practical Immunopathology of the Skin, by *Bruce R. Smoller,* MD, *2002*

PRACTICAL IMMUNOPATHOLOGY OF THE SKIN

By

BRUCE R. SMOLLER, MD

*Departments of Pathology and Dermatology,
University of Arkansas for Medical Sciences,
Little Rock, AR*

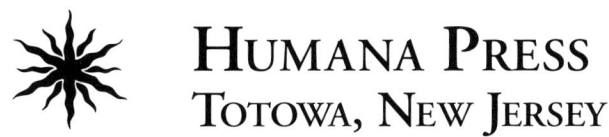

HUMANA PRESS
TOTOWA, NEW JERSEY

© 2002 Humana Press Inc.
999 Riverview Drive, Suite 208
Totowa, New Jersey 07512

www.humanapress.com

Production Editor: Jessica Jannicelli.
Cover design by Patricia F. Cleary.

Cover Illustration:Chapter 2, Fig. 2. Aminoethylcarbazol produces a bright red end product that contrasts with the blue counterstain. Further, this reagent allows distinction from endogenous melanin that may be present in the tissue sections.

This publication is printed on acid-free paper. ∞
ANSI Z39.48-1984 (American National Standards Institute) Permanence of Paper for Printed Library Materials.

For additional copies, pricing for bulk purchases, and/or information about other Humana titles, contact Humana at the above address or at any of the following numbers: Tel.: 973-256-1699; Fax: 973-256-8341; E-mail: humana@humanapr.com or visit our website: http://humanapress.com

Printed in the United States of America.   10 9 8 7 6 5 4 3 2 1
Library of Congress Cataloging-in-Publication Data

Smoller, Bruce R.
   Practical immunopathology of the skin / by Bruce R. Smoller
      p. ; cm. -- (Current clinical pathology)
   Includes bibliographical references and index.
   ISBN 1-58829-149-9 (alk. paper)
   1. Skin--Diseases--Immunodiagnosis. 2. Immunoenzyme technique. I. Title. II. Series.
   [DNLM: 1. Skin--immunology. 2. Skin--pathology. 3. Antibodies. 4. Biological
   Markers. 5. Immunologic Techniques. WR 105 S666p 2003]
   RL97 . S68 2003
   616,5'079--dc21
                                                          2002027342

PREFACE

Practical Immunopathology of the Skin begins with a discussion of the science behind immunopathology and an explanation of the immunoperoxidase technique and its most frequently used modifications. Issues of tissue preparation, antigen retrieval techniques, and pitfalls that occur in the laboratory will be addressed.

Following the introductory sections dealing with technique and laboratory issues, a working library of antibody probes is introduced. The antibodies are arbitrarily divided into categories based upon the types of cells they help to characterize. However, as is the case with any categorization system, there is some overlap, and antibodies might fit easily into more than one category. In these situations, I opted for the location that fits best into my strategy scheme when deciding upon an antibody profile. For instance, anti-cytokeratin 20 is an anti-cytokeratin antibody, but is used most commonly to identify Merkel cell carcinomas, neuroendocrine tumors. Thus, I have chosen to discuss this antibody in the chapter addressing markers of neuroendocrine cells. For each antibody discussed, I offer a small introductory paragraph that provides a general overview of the known information about the targeted antigen and its role in cellular function. I then progress to a discussion of the diagnostic utility of the probe, attempting to highlight the uses and potentially confounding features of each. When available, sensitivities and specificities for these markers in identifying various neoplasms are cited. More specific technical aspects of each antibody, including any personal experiences we have encountered with the antibodies in our laboratory, are mentioned. The discussion of each potential probe is summarized with a terse statement of its potential uses in a diagnostic dermatopathology laboratory.

The final section of *Practical Immunopathology of the Skin* is a series of vignettes taken from my practice. I have selected a range of real cases designed to exemplify a strategy for the employment of immunopathology. For each scenario, clinical history is presented along with the photomicrographs from the original, routinely stained microscopic sections. These sections are sometimes less than ideal and they have been chosen for this reason in order to fully demonstrate the benefits of immunopathology. A differential diagnosis is constructed based upon the available information and a strategy for solving the diagnostic dilemma is presented in tabular form. Results of the staining procedures are presented and there is a concluding statement explaining some specifics of the case.

It is my hope to keep the book on the level of a practical, "user's manual" rather than that of an in-depth, scientific treatise on the subject. I believe that the theoretical aspects of immunopathology are well covered by other authors and I will make frequent reference to these works throughout the book.

Bruce R. Smoller, MD

ACKNOWLEDGMENTS

There are many people who are important to me and to whom I am deeply indebted. Without them, I would not have had the opportunity to write this book. I want to sincerely thank my histology technicians, Vicky Givens and Lori Talley, whose work is reflected in the photomicrographs throughout this volume. I also want to thank Vicky for her helpful comments and critical appraisals of my writings. She is a terrific "fact-checker." I would like to express my gratitude to Drs. Laura Lamps, David Parham, and Lija Joseph who contributed some of the immunostained cases that I photographed for this book. I also would like to thank the many dermatology and pathology residents with whom I have had the privilege of working over the past years. It is at their request that I embarked upon this task.

Finally, and most importantly, I wish to thank my wonderful wife, Laura, and my two children, Gabey and Jason, for permitting me the time for this undertaking. They are unfailingly supportive and I never cease to appreciate and love them.

CONTENTS

I | INTRODUCTION

1 Overview

What is Immunopathology?

Immunopathology is a scientific discipline that enables diagnostic pathologists to visualize cellular characteristics not apparent by routine histochemical stains. Immunopathologic techniques have evolved over the past twenty years and continue to evolve at a rapid pace. The scientific methods behind the process have remained largely stable, but techniques designed to enhance sensitivity and specificity are being discovered continuously. In addition, the immunologic probes available to diagnosticians are forever changing and becoming progressively more sophisticated.

What is Immunoperoxidase?

Immunoperoxidase is, quite simply, a scientific technique that enables pathologists to visualize cellular antigens. It is defined more precisely as the technique that specifically uses a peroxidase-based amplification and visualization sequence. However, within current general usage, the term has become largely synonymous with each of the modifications of the technique that accomplish the same functions, such as the avidin-biotin complexing technique or an alkaline phosphatase-based technique.

What are the Goals of Immunopathology?

Immunopathology should serve to allow the diagnostician the ability to visualize cellular characteristics not seen with routine histochemical stains. The identification of cellular features helps with determining the differentiation or cell of origin giving rise to the process being examined. This information can then be used to affix a name to a process. While establishing a diagnosis may ultimately lead to a "benign" or "malignant" diagnosis, the immunopathology findings do not directly give rise to this prognosis. The findings can only serve to identify cell types, and these findings *must* be interpreted within the context of clinical and histologic features. Immu-

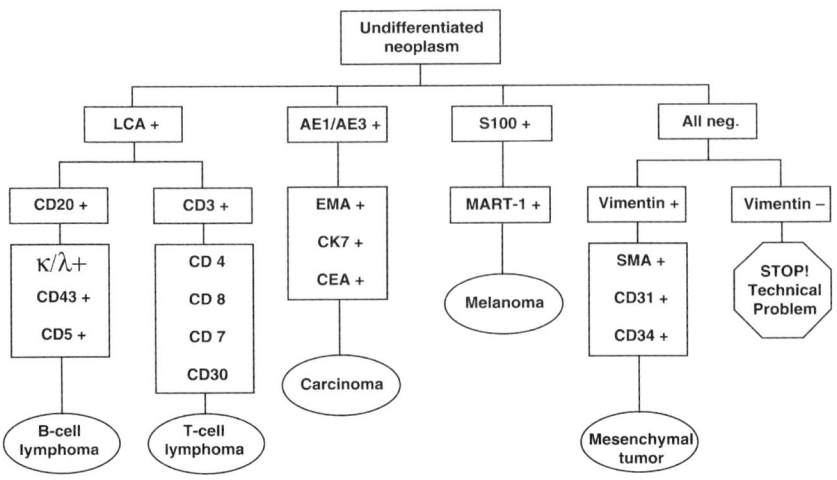

Fig. 1. Sample algorithmic method for working up an undifferentiated neoplasm in the skin.

nopathology should never be used to make a determination of benign or malignant. At this time, there are no markers identified that can serve this function.

When Should Immunoperoxidase be Used?

Immunoperoxidase methods should be used in situations where simple examination of the routine histologic sections cannot resolve the types of cells involved in a process. In all cases, every attempt should be made to establish a diagnosis, or at least to construct a narrow, reasonable differential diagnosis prior to employing immunoperoxidase. Only after this analysis has been completed can a rational strategy for immunopathology be devised. One such strategy is outlined schematically in Fig. 1. As this flow chart demonstrates, an algorithmic logic should be used in the selection of immunoreagents for examination. In Fig. 1, the diagnostic pathologist is confronted with a slide in which there are undifferentiated tumor cells that cannot be further classified on routine sections. An antibody panel designed to classify the neoplasm into one of several large categories is selected, followed by a secondary level of antibodies chosen based upon the results of the first round of immunostains. A tertiary level of antibodies follows in some cases. In this particular case, the pathologist selected an initial panel of antibodies that served to identify a tumor as epithelial, mesenchymal, or hematopoietic (a subset of mesenchymal tumors). Based upon these findings, a second set of antibodies was constructed that served to further subtype the types of cells involved in the proliferation. The pathologist also recognized the possibility of a problem with the tissue, including a plan for working up the situation in which no immunostaining was identified. This type of approach is both cost-effective and serves to minimize irrelevant immunostains that could confound interpretation. More specific examples are discussed in Part III of this book.

Where is Immunoperoxidase Performed?

Immunoperoxidase laboratories exist within virtually all university-based pathology departments. Most large private surgical pathology or dermatopathology laboratories also have immunoperoxidase sections. The technique has become an essential component of diagnostic pathology, and most diagnostic pathologists do not believe that they can practice the specialty without immunostains. In some smaller groups, pathologists refer cases requiring immunostaining to larger laboratories or even regional immunopathology referral centers. Wherever the immunostaining procedures are performed, it is essential that the laboratory be fully accredited and in compliance with federal and regional regulatory agencies. This regulation is of vital importance for patient care. The procedures involved in immunostaining are complex, and the reagents used are dangerous and must be used correctly and judiciously. Failure to comply strictly with standardized laboratory techniques can result in spurious laboratory results and aberrant diagnoses.

Who Oversees the Immunopathology Laboratory?

As mentioned previously, immunopathology laboratories exist under the auspices of a larger diagnostic pathology laboratory. In most cases, a licensed physician trained in laboratory medicine (i.e., surgical pathologist and dermatopathologist) functions as the laboratory director. This physician generally entrusts the daily direction of the laboratory to a laboratory supervisor who may function as an administrator or as an immunopathology technician. The responsibility for maintaining quality control and quality assurance within the laboratory falls upon these two individuals. It is also essential that

laboratory directors maintain knowledge of current rules and regula-
tions for laboratories and keep abreast of the rapidly changing
advances in the field.

When is the Decision Made to Use Immunopathologic Examinations?

The answer to this question has changed over the past decade and
will continue to be modified, as there are new developments in the
science behind the technique. In its infancy, antibodies recognized
antigens found only on cells in unfixed tissue samples. During this
time, physicians made decisions about the necessity of immunostaining at the time of the biopsy. Pathologists set aside frozen tissue
for immunostaining prior to review of the routine histologic sections.
Needless to say, this was a great impediment to the widespread imple-
mentation of the technique. Over the past decade, scientists have
developed antibodies that recognize an ever-increasing number of
antigens that survive routine processing techniques. Further, investigators have described a wide range of antigen retrieval techniques that
unmask antigens previously hidden by fixation. Most recently, scientific research has provided diagnosticians with antibodies that recognize lymphocyte surface antigens in fixed tissue. At the present time,
decisions about if and when to perform immunostains can almost
invariably be made after reviewing initial histologic sections. There is
no longer need for specially processed or unfixed tissue.

Who Should Interpret Immunostaining Results?

Immunopathology is a complex medical test and should be interpreted by a trained and experienced physician. While in some laboratories, the final result may be reported simply as "positive" or
"negative," interpretation of the data is not so straightforward. It is
essential to know if all of the controls worked adequately during the
testing of the slide in question. It is also important to know the quality
of the staining. For instance, is the colorimetric precipitate located
within nuclei or the cytoplasm of cells? For some antibodies, only
nuclear staining should be considered truly "positive." It is important
to be able to discount any apparent staining in areas of necrosis, or at
the edges of the specimen.

Physicians should not use immunostaining results as the sole tool
to make a diagnosis. Data attained from the immunostaining should

be used along with the information gleaned from the routine histologic sections. Further, this information must be interpreted within the clinical context of the patient as a whole before arriving at a final diagnosis. Thus, it is the responsibility of any physician to understand the role of immunostaining results in arriving at a final diagnosis. Even for dermatologists who do not interpret their own histology slides or immunostaining results, it is important that they understand the general principles of immunopathology, the possible limitations and pitfalls of the technique, and the sources for possible erroneous interpretation.

What are the Limitations to Using Immunoperoxidase?

As is the case with any laboratory test, immunopathology is not an exact process. There are limitations of sensitivity and specificity inherent in the technique. Problems with sensitivity can arise on account of the primary antibodies or owing to problems at any point along the procedure itself. Problems with fixation, antigen retrieval, incubation times, antibody concentrations, and other reagents can all limit the sensitivity of immunoreactions. Similarly, these same parameters can alter the specificity of any antibody (some of which have at least some cross-reactivity with other antigens). Thus, it is vital that results of immunostaining be interpreted in the context of the entire case, including the routine histologic sections as well as any clinical information.

It is most important at all times to remember that immunolabeling should never be used to determine benign from malignant directly. This distinction may become apparent once a cell type has been identified and added to the remainder of the case scenario, but on its own, this is not an appropriate use for immunopathology.

2 Immunoperoxidase
The Technique

Tissue Preparation
Fixation

Tissue specimens must be fixed properly in order to attain adequate histologic sections. There are currently many types of fixative available for this purpose. The various types of fixative have different methods of stabilizing the tissues, thus resulting in different effects on the immunopathology process. Some of the commercially available fixatives are alcohol-based, while others contain heavy metals as the main operative component. However, virtually all diagnostic dermatopathology laboratories use a formaldehyde-based fixative for routine tissue fixation. These fixatives are readily available, relatively inexpensive, and provide good fixation for most tissues and clinical situations. As other fixatives such as mercury-based, picric acid, and alcohol-based fixatives are not widely used in dermatopathology, their inherent problems pertaining to immunopathology will not be discussed in this volume. For more specific information addressing these specific issues, the readers are referred to more generalized textbooks of immunopathology *(1)*. It is important to be aware of the different problems if other fixatives are used. In many places, mercuric acid fixatives are used for biopsies of suspected cutaneous lymphoma, especially when hematopathology laboratories are involved in the initial work-up.

The most widely used fixative in dermatopathology laboratories consists of 4% formalin solution, made by diluting 40% formaldehyde into a 10% solution with neutralized, buffered saline. Fortunately, formalin fixation allows for excellent immunoreactivity with a large number of diagnostically useful antibodies. Formalin works by crosslinking proteins within the cells of the tissue by forming hydroxymethyl groups *(2)*. This serves to "mask" some of the cellular antigens, but these effects can be reversed during the immunoperoxidase procedures.

Formalin penetrates tissue specimens relatively slowly. Ideal fixation is essential for optimal immunostaining results. Fixation time is therefore a very important variable to consider in tissue preparation. A 3-mm punch biopsy of skin takes approx 8 h to fully fix, and this is the ideal fixation time for subsequent immunostaining procedures. Overfixation can also result in diminished tissue immunogenicity *(1)*. For this reason, it is usually not advisable to fix tissue sections for greater than 24 h. As with many chemical reagents, newly mixed formalin solution would ideally be created each day. As the buffered formalin solution ages, immunostaining results may be adversely affected. However, in most laboratories, the formalin supply is kept current by rapid turnover of specimen bottles, rather than the daily creation of fresh formalin solution. For this reason, the age of the fixative used is rarely a factor in the immunopathology laboratory. It is important to maintain a near neutral pH for the solution, as acidic pHs can diminish immunostaining. (Extensive decalcification with acetic acid may decrease tissue antigenicity, though this procedure is seldom used in dermatopathology.)

Many immunomarkers do not recognize antigens in tissue following formalin fixation. However, few of these are in use in routine diagnostic dermatopathology. Previously, altered antigen recognition occurred with many of the antibodies directed against lymphocyte surface antigens. However, antibodies have been developed that can recognize these same (or related) antigens in formalin-fixed tissue sections. Other antibodies such as keratin-specific anticytokeratin antibodies are now being developed that can recognize specific cytokeratins in fixed tissue sections.

A little used, but valuable, technique is microwave tissue fixation. Subjecting fresh tissue immersed in a dilute aldehyde solution to microwave irradiation allows rapid fixation with good preservation of morphology and preservation of antigens. In many cases, antibodies can recognize these antigens, without the pretreatment procedures such as enzymatic digestion (*see* the following section) sometimes required with formalin-fixed tissue *(3)*.

Paraffin Embedding

Virtually all diagnostic dermatopathology laboratories generate microscope slides from tissue sections embedded in paraffin. This part of the processing involves placing the fixed tissue sections into paraffin that has been heated to a liquid state and then cooling the properly embedded tissue specimen back to a solid state. While varying the temperatures and types of paraffin used in this process affect immunolabeling results, in most laboratories, the embedding process is standardized. If these conditions remain constant, subsequent immunolabeling techniques can be established within the laboratory to maximize staining results. Thus, this step in the tissue processing rarely contributes significantly to the quality of immunostaining results.

Immunostaining can be performed adequately and reproducibly on archived tissue sections. There is a suggestion that at least some antibodies lose some sensitivity when used on blocks that have been stored for long periods. However, antigen retrieval techniques (described in the Enzymatic Epitope Retrieval section) can often enhance the sensitivities. In most cases, this is not a significant problem, though it should be kept in mind when attempting to evaluate staining results on older cases.

Slide Preparation

Immunolabeling techniques require tissue sections to be placed on special types of glass slides. Because of the repeated incubation and washing steps required in the various processes (*see* below), paraffin-embedded tissue sections often become dislodged and wash off of ordinary glass microscope slides. There are several types of specially prepared microscope slides designed to overcome this problem. Slides coated with poly-L-lysine, or positively charged slides can be purchased that are much more effective at retaining tissue sections throughout the immunostaining procedure. Coating ordinary slides with a slight film of common glue will also solve the problem, but this step requires more effort of the laboratory personnel. In addition, the quality control will not be as uniform with locally produced "sticky" slides.

Drying the slides is an additional step required to assure that tissue sections remain attached to the slides. After cutting the sections to be immunolabeled, the slides are placed in a conventional oven (at <60°C) for at least an hour. Most laboratories heat the slides for longer than this. There is marked variation from laboratory to laboratory at this point in the specimen preparation, but some type of slide drying is considered essential in most laboratories.

Techniques for Antigen Visualization

There are many different laboratory techniques that have been developed that are designed to enable the visualization of cellular antigens. All of the techniques are variations on the theme of an indirect immunopathologic method. Over the past 25 yr, investigators have continued to modify this basic process in order to maximize sensitivity and specificity while keeping background staining to a minimum.

The basic laboratory strategy is depicted in Diagram 1. A commercially prepared "nonlabeled" primary antibody from a nonhuman source directed against a specific antibody found in human tissue (i.e., rabbit anti-human S100 protein) is put onto a glass slide containing tissue to be examined. The slide is then washed in a buffering solution. Antibody that is bound to the specifically sought antigen will remain on the tissue sections and all unbound antibodies will be washed away. A second antibody directed against immunoglobulins from the first animal, created in different species from the first animal (i.e., goat anti-rabbit IgG) is placed on the tissue sections with a large excess of antibody. Following an incubation period, the slide is again washed with a buffer solution, rinsing away the unbound antibodies. These secondary antibodies are labeled with a reagent such as peroxidase to allow visualization of the developing antibody complex. This method enables a wide range of unlabeled primary antibodies to be used in conjunction with one (or several) secondary antibodies that not are specific for any primary human antigens, but simply react with immunoglobulin from a nonhuman source. These "labeled" antibodies are ultimately enzymatically linked to the colorimetric end product that is seen by the interpreter. The modifications in the immunopathology methods are largely concerned with the bridging (secondary) antibodies and the end-point precipitates. There are also several points during which "blocking" steps can be added to decrease background staining, especially important with the secondary antibodies.

Diagram 1A–C. *(opposite page)* Sample protocol for immunoperoxidase staining method. **(A)** Cells within tissue sections are incubated with a mouse anti-human (i.e., S100 protein) antibody (M). **(B)** Excess, unbound mouse anti-human antibodies are rinsed off with buffer, leaving only antibody specifically bound to the human cellular antigen. **(C)** The tissue sections are then incubated with rabbit anti-mouse immunoglobulin antibodies (R).

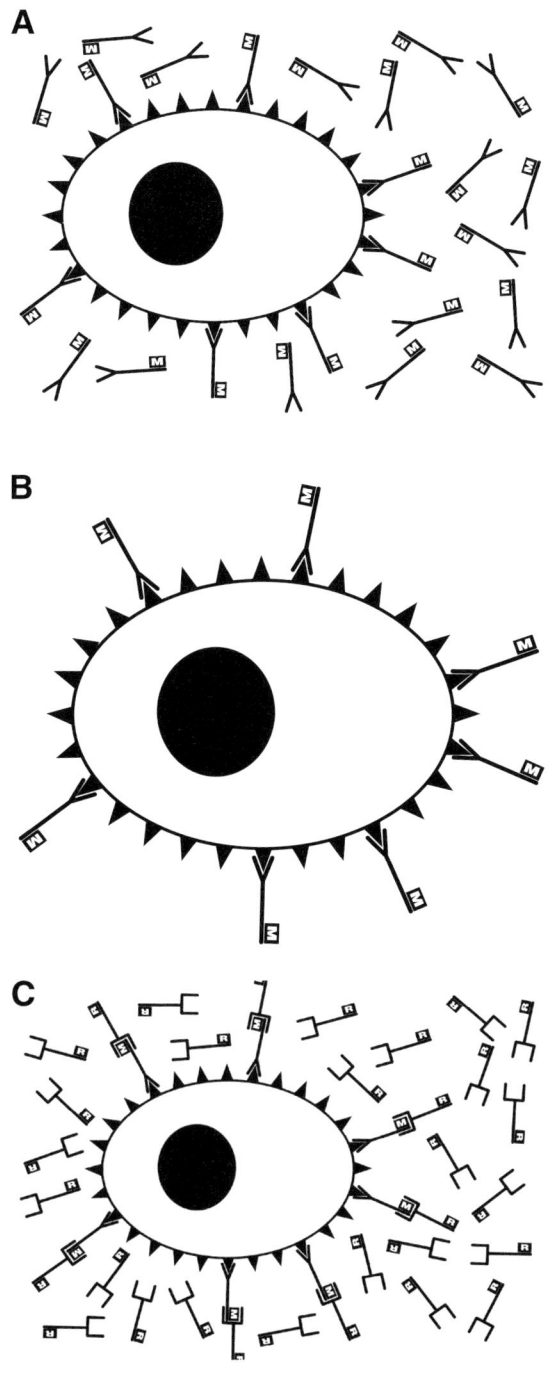

Diagram 1A–C.

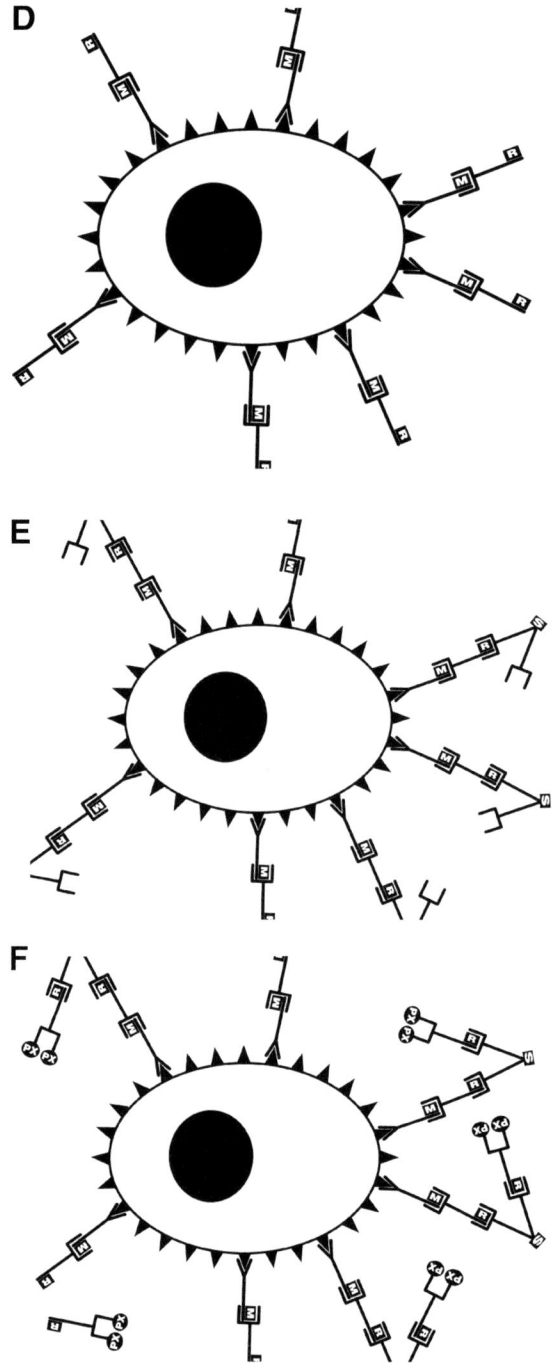

Diagram 1D–F.

Diagram 1D–F. *(opposite page)* Excess, unbound rabbit antibodies are rinsed off, leaving only rabbit antibody that specifically bound to the mouse immunoglobulins. **(E)** Tissue sections are incubated with swine anti-rabbit antibodies (S), the so-called bridge antibodies. (Excess, unbound swine antibodies are rinsed, not shown). **(F)** A preformed peroxidase anti-peroxidase complex (PX), formed on rabbit antibodies are incubated with the tissue sections and bind to unbound receptors on the swine antibodies. (Excess, unbound conjugated rabbit antibodies are rinsed, not shown.)

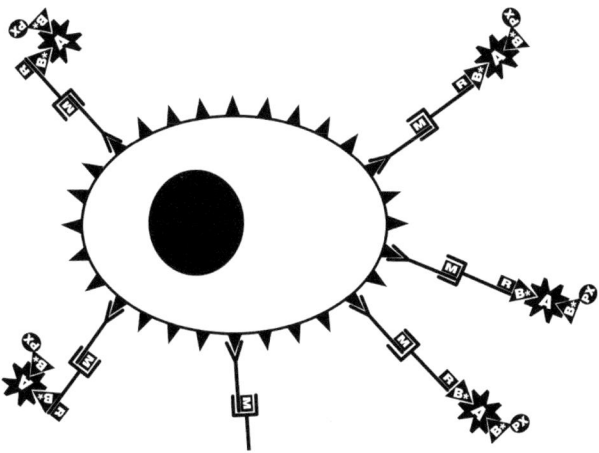

Diagram 2. Avidin-biotin-peroxidase method. The diagram shows the final stage in the avidin-biotin-peroxidase modification of the immunopathology technique. Specific mouse anti-human (i.e. desmin) antibodies are bound to a cell. A rabbit-anti-mouse IgG is complexed with biotin and binds to the bound mouse immunoglobulin. The tissue sections are incubated with avidin and with biotin conjugated to peroxidase. (Intermediate steps are not shown, but are similar in principle to those demonstrated in Diagram 1.)

The most commonly employed immunopathology technique at this time is the biotin-streptavidin immunoperoxidase complex (B-SA) method (Diagram 2). The standard, unlabeled primary antibody is applied to tissue sections and unbound antibody washed off the sections. In this modification of the immunostaining technique, the secondary antibody directed against the species from which the primary antibody is derived is labeled on one end with the vitamin biotin. Following an incubation with the tissue section, excess, unbound antibody is washed away. Streptavidin, a 60-kD analog of avidin with multiple high-affinity binding sites for biotin, is added to the tissue sections, followed by biotinylated peroxidase. This complex is incubated with the tissue sections containing primary antibody and biotinylated secondary antibody. This incubation takes place in conditions of great streptavidin excess, thus enabling the formation of large peroxidase complexes. The final colorimetric precipitate proceeds in a manner identical to the original peroxidase antiperoxidase method. The avidin-biotin-immunoperoxidase method is thought by some to be more sensitive than earlier methods (4).

Colorimetric End-Products
Diaminobenzidine (DAB)

The most commonly used colorimetric precipitate used in immunostaining laboratories is diaminobenzidine. This reagent yields a strong brown precipitate that is easily visualized with any type of counterstain (or without) on tissue sections, serving as an oxidant for the horseradish peroxidase- H_2O_2 complex (Fig. 1). It has the advantage of being relatively sensitive and permanent. The precipitate does not fade over time. One disadvantage is that the compound is a carcinogen, but this is not a major concern for most laboratories, as it is believed that the risks from exposure to DAB are relatively small. There are a variety of modifications that can be used to enhance the intensity of the DAB end product. Increasing the incubation time of the tissue section with the DAB and hydrogen peroxidase to form the precipitate will increase the staining intensity, but often will increase background staining in parallel. Incorporation of heavy metals into the DAB mixture will increase the signal:noise ratio effectively. Copper sulfate is the most commonly used heavy metal, but osmium tetroxide, cobalt chloride, and nickel have also been used to enhance the DAB intensity (5).

Aminoethylcarbazol (AEC)

Another frequently used chromagen is aminoethylcarbazol (AEC). AEC produces a bright red color that is easy to visualize and to photograph. It also has the advantage of not being carcinogenic. However, the major drawback to AEC is that the color tends to fade over time. The intensity of the staining decreases over months, and the chromagen tends to bleed into the surrounding tissue. Thus, the slides cannot be regarded as permanent records. In our laboratory, AEC has repeatedly proven to yield less sensitive results than DAB.

One great advantage to AEC over DAB is when immunostaining is required for cells that contain abundant melanin and/or hemosid-

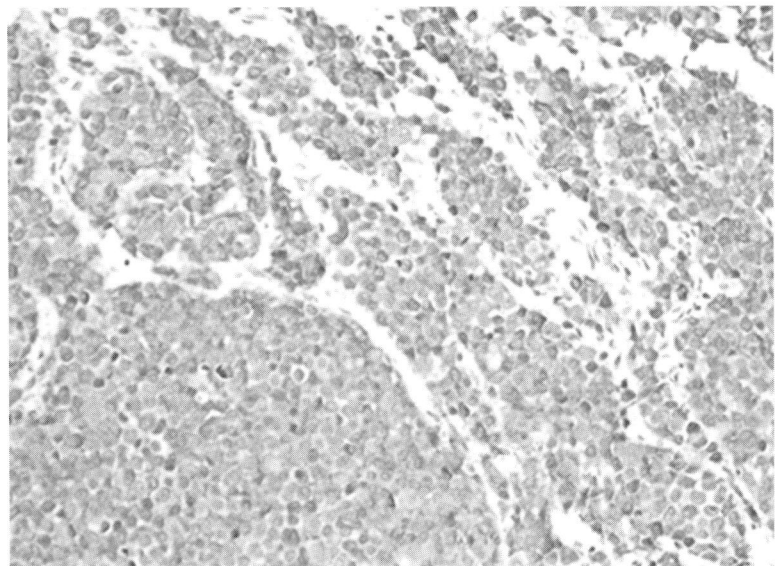

Fig. 1. Diaminobenzidine (DAB) yields a dark brown precipitate that contrasts with the blue counterstain. (*See* color plate 1 appearing in the insert following p. 22.)

erin (Fig. 2). It can be quite difficult to distinguish immunostaining from these endogenous pigments when DAB is used as the chromagen, as all appear brown on tissue sections. However, the AEC provides a nice contrast between a red, positive immunostaining reaction and endogenous brown pigment. In some cases, we have found the use of AEC as a chromagen helpful in detecting true staining in heavily pigmented cells. (Another technique is to bleach the tissue sections with H_2O_2 prior to immunolabeling. The S100 protein will survive this pre-treatment, though antigens recognized by MART-1 and HMB-45 do not survive very well.)

Alkaline Phosphatase

Some laboratories prefer an alkaline phosphatase-based colorimetric system. This system yields a brilliant red end product. It is not as widely used as the systems described earlier.

Antibodies

A primary antibody that identifies a given antigen is applied to tissue sections. This primary antibody is developed in an animal other than a human being and is directed against an antigen found on human

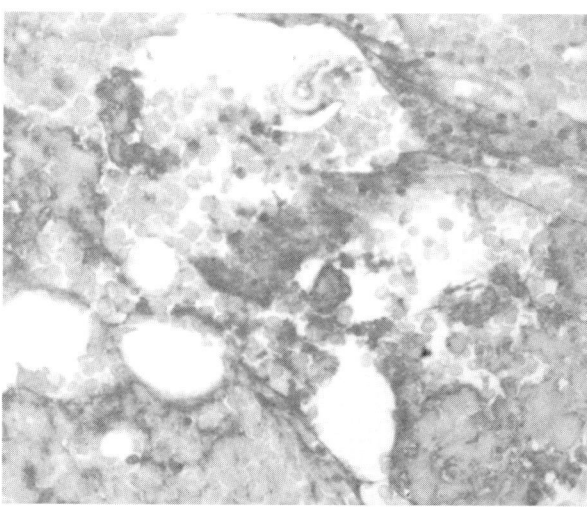

Fig. 2. Aminoethylcarbazol produces a bright red end product that contrasts with the blue counterstain. Further, this reagent allows distinction from endogenous melanin that may be present in the tissue sections. (*See* color plate 2 appearing in the insert following p. 22.)

cells. These antibodies can be either monoclonal or polyclonal and are produced by a variety of methods. Monoclonal antibodies are more specific than are polyclonal antibodies, but are more likely to be adversely affected by fixation problems *(6)*. Polyclonal antibodies tend to have higher binding affinities for specific antigens than do their monoclonal counterpart *(7)*. Most commonly, hybridoma technology using mice is the method used for generating monoclonal antibodies. In diagnostic dermatopathology, only commercially available antibodies are used. Thus, an in-depth discussion on the methods for developing new antibodies is outside the scope of this volume. It is important to realize, however, that every antibody has its own specificity and sensitivity. Each manufacturer's antibodies have unique staining properties. It is imperative to learn the behavior pattern of each antibody before employing it in routine clinical work, both in the printed materials supplied by the manufacturers as well as performance of the antibodies in the laboratory using them. Extensive testing should be performed on each new antibody in order to develop maximum performance in each individual laboratory. It is not sufficient simply to use the manufacturer's suggested protocols, as performance varies widely from location to location.

A secondary antibody directed against the primary antibody is required for all the antigen detection methods described. These antibodies are most commonly anti-immunoglobulin antibodies directed against immunoglobulins that comprise the primary antibody. These secondary antibodies must be somewhat species-specific and cannot react with human tissue. Several companies now produce secondary antibody cocktails that recognize immunoglobulins from several species, and can be used with a large number of primary antibodies.

Commercially available antibodies have a recommended shelf life. It is essential that outdated antibodies be discarded and not used for diagnostic purposes. In addition to being a laboratory regulation enforced by several accreditation boards, results obtained with outdated antibodies may not be reproducible, leading to erroneous results and compromising patient care.

Controls

As with every laboratory test, it is imperative that appropriate controls be performed with each immunostaining procedure. Several types of controls are essential in order to permit the accurate interpretation of immunostaining results. Controls take the form of internal controls and external controls. For immunostaining procedures, probably the most important controls are internal. For each antibody tested, it is imperative that cell types that are expected to label with an antibody demonstrate the appropriate positive staining reaction on the tissue being examined (a positive internal control). It is equally important that cell types that are not expected to react with a given antibody are appropriately negative on the tissue section being examined (negative internal control). These controls provide the information that the tissue section has been fixed in a manner that preserves the antigen in question. It also provides the information that the staining procedure worked. Further, it allows the interpreter to see the specific antibody working as expected.

In addition to the internal controls, most laboratories have several different types of external controls that are run with each immunolabeling procedure. In order to assure that the immunostaining procedure worked appropriately, tissue sections taken from a specimen known to be reactive with a given antibody are run in parallel with the sections being tested diagnostically. This tissue serves as a positive external control. In many laboratories, a standardized "sausage-like" tissue section comprised of a wide range of cell types serves as the positive external control. This type of tissue specimen can be prepared locally or purchased commercially. If the external control specimen stains appropriately but there is no staining whatsoever on the experimental tissue (including cells that should label with the antibody), it is likely that there is a problem with antigen recognition on the tissue to be examined. This result might suggest over- or underfixation, or several other problems. Additional antigen retrieval steps (*see* the Enzymatic Epitope Retrieval section) might be indicated. In addition, a negative external control specimen may be run. In most cases, this is a tissue section that undergoes all of the immunostaining procedural steps except that instead of the primary antibody being tested, an irrelevant antibody (or normal immune serum) is used. Any staining in this section can thus be regarded as nonspecific staining. Should this be significant, extreme caution should be used in interpreting the specimen being examined.

It has been suggested that the use of a ubiquitous antibody such as vimentin is helpful in assuring the antigenicity of each tissue section examined *(8)*. Vimentin labels cells that are present in virtually every specimen examined. Lack of any staining with vimentin on a slide suggests the likelihood of decreased antigen preservation and should preclude interpretation of immunostaining results.

While there are many other types of controls that can be undertaken, in most situations these are the only controls run during the immunostaining procedures. All control tissues should be examined prior to examining the test specimen so that the immunostaining results can be interpreted fairly.

Automation

The last decade has witnessed the development of automated slide stainers capable of performing immunopathologic procedures. The great advantage to these machines is their reproducibility. Preprogramming a set of incubation times and antibody dilutions essentially eliminates run-to-run variations. There are many commercially available immunostainers currently available. Each of these has its own strengths and weaknesses, and allows the laboratory personnel varying levels of control and abilities to modify individual programs.

For the usual dermatopathology laboratory that performs at least a moderate volume of immunostains, automated immunostainers have become a cost-effective part of the laboratory resources. An automated slide stainer has built-in computer technology that enables the operator to program protocols for a large number of antibodies. This is done at the time that any new antibody is brought into the laboratory and added to diagnostic work-ups. Each of the antibodies is initially analyzed in the laboratory, and the protocol for optimizing each one is established and programmed into the immunostainer prior to performing the tests on any cases. Optimization generally requires parameters such as dilutions, incubation times, and pretreatment conditions. While individual cases may require some manual "tweaking" of this program, the protocol for each antibody ideally is established to allow for best results in the vast majority of cases. The immunotechnologist prepares the tissue sections (including any required pretreatments described elsewhere) and places the entire day's slides to be immunostained onto the machine. (Most machines can hold up to 40–50 slides for a single run.) The immunostainer is preprogrammed for the day's run, taking great care to correctly correlate the slide number with the required antibodies. Once the prepared slides have been placed onto the slide racks and the computer appropriately programmed, the immunostaining procedures automatically occur. The stainer simultaneously performs the individualized protocols for each of the antibodies requested, varying the incubation times, dilutions and other parameters as preprogrammed. However, the protocol for each primary antibody remains essentially identical from run to run. The immunostainer thus provides standardization and is a labor saving device.

Additional assets to automated slide stainers include the ability to perform routine histochemical stains, direct immunofluorescence procedures, and in some cases, many of the steps required for *in situ* hybridization and polymerase chain reactions (PCR).

Modifications in Antigen Retrieval
Enzymatic Epitope Retrieval

Formalin fixation, paraffin embedding, and other tissue processing techniques alter tissue in many ways. Cellular proteins are crosslinked and masked. In some cases, this prevents primary anti-

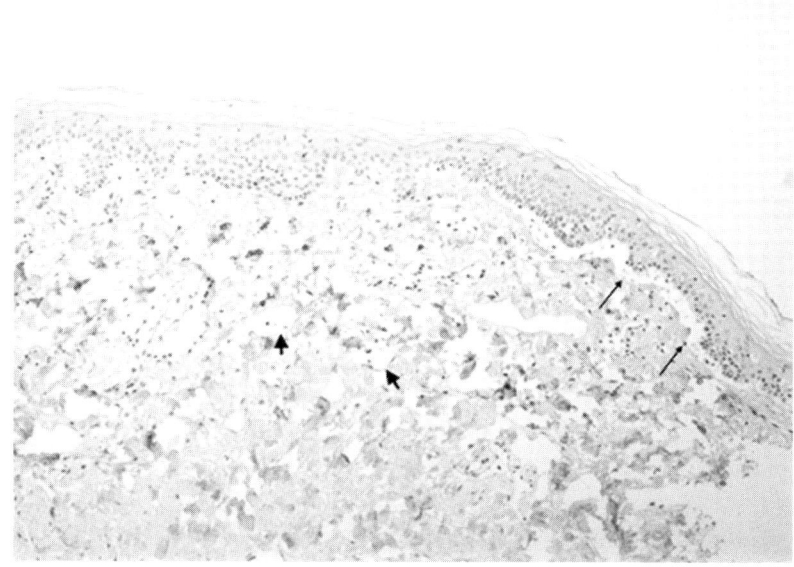

Fig. 3. Enzymatic pretreatment may result in loss of morphologic detail.

bodies from recognizing the specific cellular antigens. Overfixation in formalin can be partially reversed with the use of enzymatic digestion. Protease digestion unmasks some crosslinked immunoreactive sites and may be necessary to maximize performance of some antibodies used on routinely processed tissue sections. Protease incubation is also reported to decrease nonspecific background staining *(9)*. Incubation of tissue sections with trypsin, pepsin, pronase, ficin, DNAse, or protease is often used for this purpose *(10)*. Different incubation protocols are necessary for each of the reagents, and for each antibody to be tested. Further, it is generally recommended that the longer a tissue specimen be fixed in formalin, the longer it needs to be enzymatically pretreated. In actual practice, laboratories seldom pay heed to this rule, as there is a general assumption that all skin biopsies are fixed for approximately the same amount of time in a given laboratory setting. It is only when individual immunostaining results appear that this step is varied.

The major drawback to enzymatic tissue digestion is the loss of morphologic detail (Fig. 3). Overtreatment results in extensive tissue artifacts and may preclude diagnosis. It also may result in

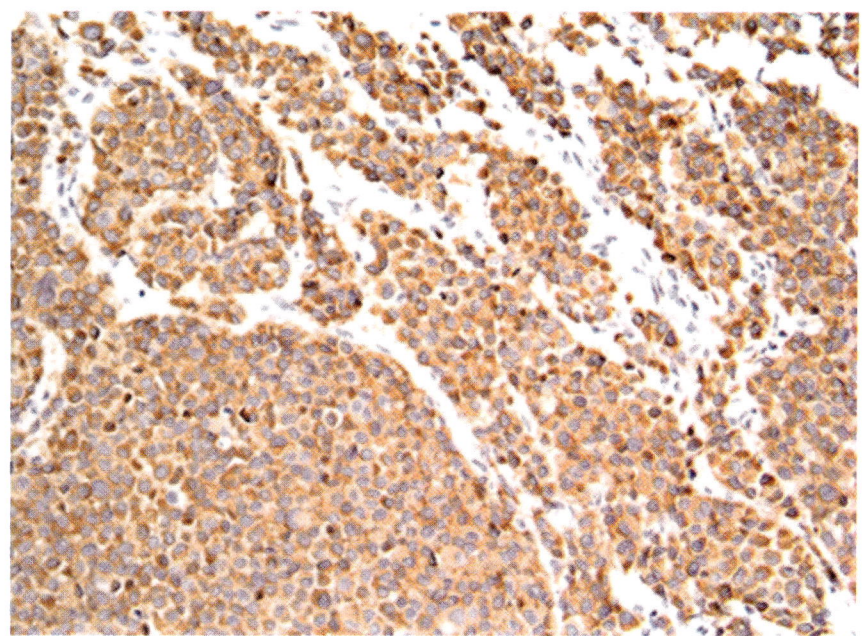

Color Plate 1, Fig. 1. (*See* discussion on p. 17.) Diaminobenzidine (DAB) yields a dark brown precipitate that contrasts with the blue counterstain.

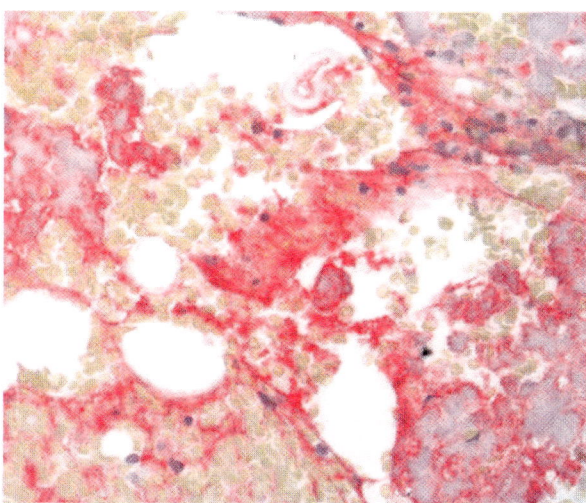

Color Plate 2, Fig. 2. (*See* discussion on p. 18.) Aminoethylcarbazol produces a bright red end product that contrasts with the blue counterstain. Further, this reagent allows distinction from endogenous melanin that may be present in the tissue sections.

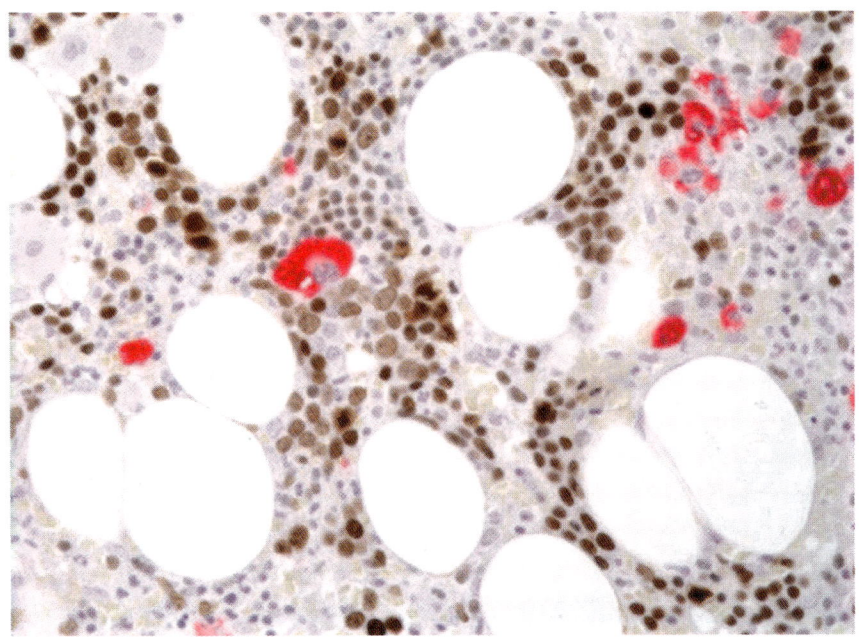

Color Plate 3, Fig. 4. (*See* discussion on p. 24.) Double labeling with kappa and lambda antibodies demonstrates separate populations of plasma cells in this specimen.

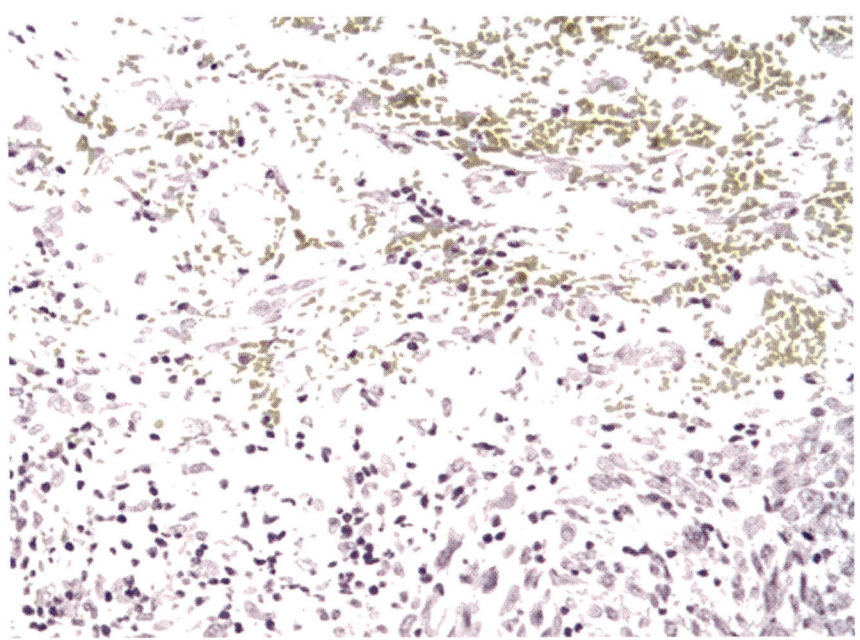

Color Plate 4, Fig. 7. (*See* discussion on p. 27.) Endogenous peroxidase activity is present in erythrocytes and granulocytes and may interfere with interpretation.

increased non-specific staining by fragmenting antigens into smaller antigenic fragments found on many cells other than the initially intended cells *(11)*.

Enzymatic epitope retrieval was the first type of antigen-enhancing technique described. Since the development of heat-induced epitope retrieval techniques, enzymatic pretreatments are used much less commonly.

Heat-Induced Epitope Retrieval

Heat-induced epitope retrieval (HIER) enhances staining with many antibodies and is required for some to recognize antigens on fixed tissue sections *(12)*. The tissue is incubated in a buffered, pre-heated solution. Water baths can be heated with pressure-cookers, microwave ovens, steamers or other types of devices. Actual protocols vary widely in terms of temperature, duration of heating and pH of the buffered solutions. However, standard protocols can be developed for routine laboratory usage that will enable generalization across most antibodies. Alkaline pHs of 8 or 9 enhance antigen retrieval, but run the risk of causing tissue damage. The literature is replete with articles explaining the relative advantages and disadvantages of shorter and longer incubation times, higher and lower incubation temperatures, methods of heating, and compositions of buffered media. In most diagnostic laboratories, however, one or several uniform methods can be established that will attain relatively good staining results with a wide range of antibodies, if not the absolute best for any given probe. For some antibodies, HIER has proven to be superior to enzymatic pretreatment. However, this is not the case with all antibodies. Gown and co-workers have published their experiences with a large number of antibodies *(13)*.

Frozen Section Immunopathology

In recent years, there has been a move to incorporate immuno-labeling into Mohs' surgery procedures in attempt to better evaluate tumor margins. Immunolabeling to identify residual pagetoid cells, be they malignant keratinocytes, melanoma cells, or tumor cells from Paget's disease is becoming more prevalent. Certainly, immunoperoxidase technology works exceedingly well on fresh, frozen tissue. However, the immunotechnician must work with an

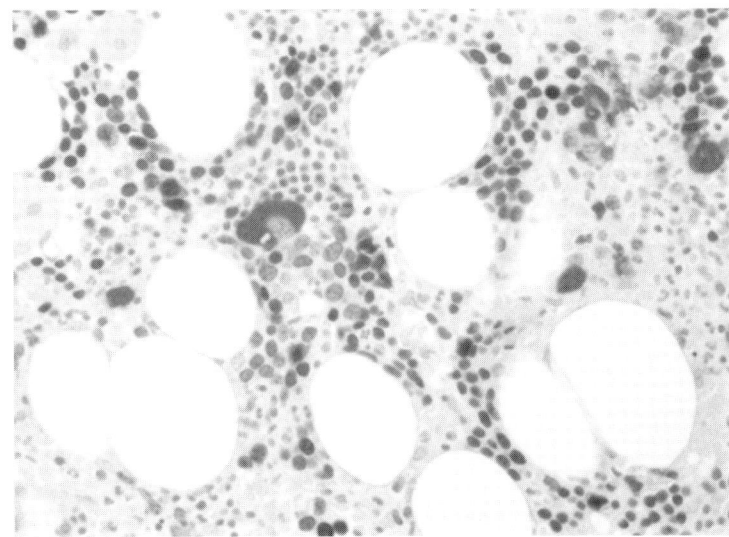

Fig. 4. Double labeling with kappa and lambda antibodies demonstrates separate populations of plasma cells in this specimen. (*See* color plate 3 appearing in the insert following p. 22.)

entirely different set of antibody dilutions and incubation times, as none of the protocols established for routinely fixed tissue will provide optimal results for frozen section analysis. Robinson has advocated the use of anti-S100 protein and HMB-45 immunostaining in order to achieve better margin control in examining narrow excisions for lentigo maligna *(14)*. Immunostains have also been used to unmask tumor cells hidden by a dense inflammatory reaction when performing frozen section examination *(15)*. A review of the use of frozen section immunoperoxidase techniques in Moh's micrographic surgery details many of the current uses for this procedure *(16)*.

Double Labeling

It is technically possible to perform double labeling with two antibodies on a single tissue section. If the primary antibodies to be used are from the same species, the immunostaining procedures are performed sequentially, varying the final colorimetric precipitate. If primary antibodies from different species are used, the immuonstaining procedures can be performed simultaneously (Fig. 4; *17*).

Table 1

Excess immunostaining	Potential solutions
Tissue dried at some point in processing	Redo making certain to keep wet at all times
Excessive enzymatic digestion	Decrease incubation time with enzymes
Excessive HIER	Decrease time of HIER incubation
Edge effect	Look at tissue away from edges
Too concentrated antibodies (primary or sencondary)	Decrease concentrations or incubation times
Too long incubations	Decrease incubation times at several steps in protocol
Too concentrated DAB	Decrease concentration of DAB or incubation time at this step
Tissue necrosis	Choose another area of slide without necrosis to interpret
Nonimmunologic binding to collagen	Find more cellular area with less collagen in tumor mass
Endogenous peroxidase not completely extinguished	Increase length of time for blocking
Overfixation	Decrease incubations or antibody concentrations

Insufficient immunostaining	Potential solutions
Tissue sections too old-deteriorated antigen preservation	Increase incubation with enzymes or HIER
Overfixation	Increase incubation with enzymes or HIER
Outdated antibodies (primary or secondary)	Try vimentin antibody to check tissue; restain with new antibodies if tissue is not the problem
Too dilute antibody concentrations (Primary or secondary)	Vary concentrations of primary and secondary antibodies (separately)
Need for antigen retrieval technique	May be required even when package insert claims otherwise
Too dilute DAB concentration	Increase concentration of DAB or incubation time

Pitfalls in the Interpretation of Immunopathology

As is the case with every laboratory test, there are many potential pitfalls in the interpretation of immunopathology results (*see* Table 1). Poor fixation can result in false negative readings if appropriate attention is not paid to internal and external controls. The presence of necro-

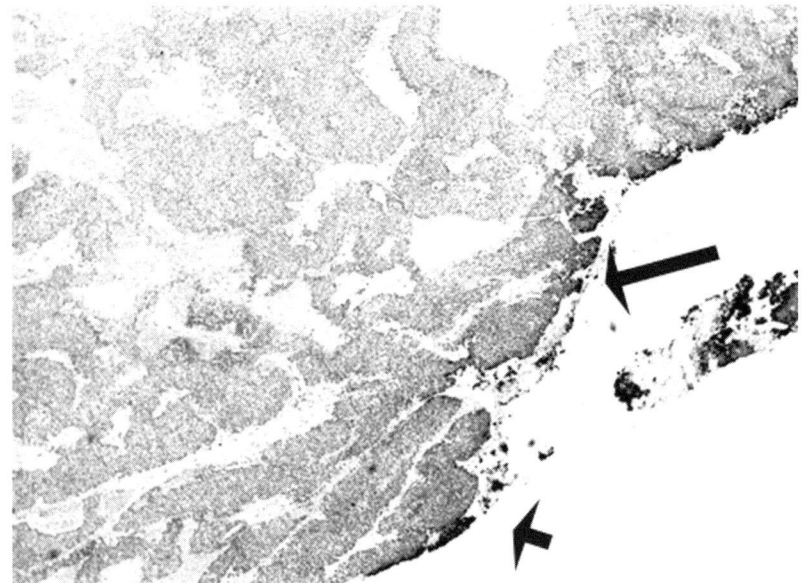

Fig. 5. The presence of necrosis contributes to a high background staining owing to nonspecific adsorption.

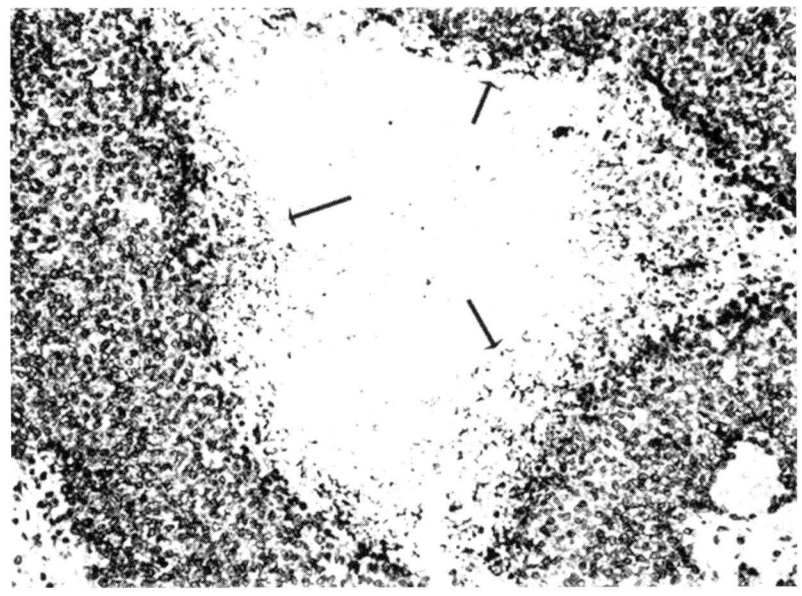

Fig. 6. An "edge effect" is often present on tissue sections. The edges of the tissue appear to be immunoreactive. This staining is not real and should be interpreted with caution.

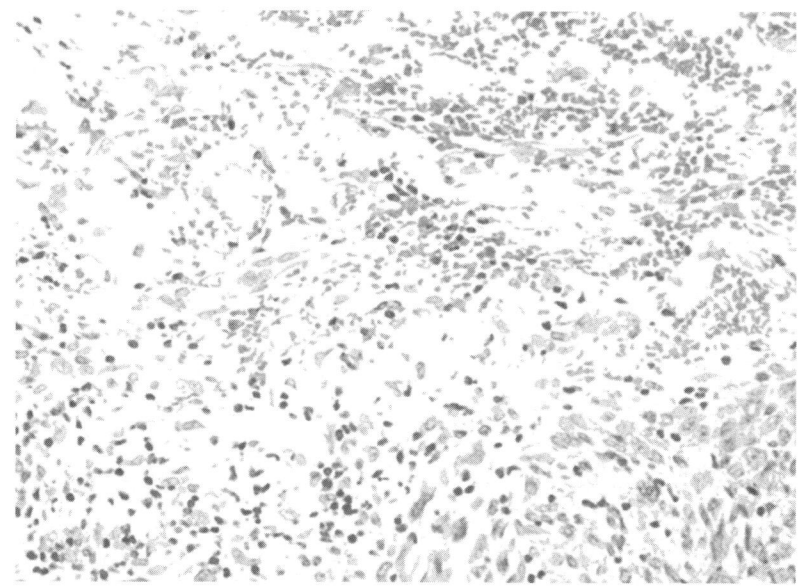

Fig. 7. Endogenous peroxidase activity is present in erythrocytes and granulocytes and may interfere with interpretation. (*See* color plate 4 appearing in the insert following p. 22.)

sis within tissue sections can result in nonspecific staining, resulting in false positive interpretations (Fig. 5). There is often an "edge-effect" such that the edges of tissue sections appear to have positive staining when none is present (Fig. 6). Similarly, drying of the tissue at any point along the staining procedure can result in excessively high backgrounds and false positive readings. Failure to extinguish endogenous peroxidase activity and erythrocytes and granulocytes can also result in increased nonspecific staining (Fig. 7). It is crucial to be aware of each of these situations prior to making a final interpretation of the immunostains.

References

1. Taylor, C. R. (1994) *Immunomicroscopy*, 2nd ed., Philadelphia: W. B. Saunders.
2. Fox, C. H., Johnson, F. B., Whiting, J., and Roller, P. P. (1985) Formaldehyde fixation. *J. Histochem. Cytochem.* **33,** 845–853.
3. Login, G. R., Schnitt, S. J., and Dvorak, A. M. (1987) Rapid microwave fixation of human tissues for light microscopic immunoperoxidase identification of diagnostically useful antigens. *Lab. Invest.* **57,** 585–591.
4. Hsu, S.-M., Raine, L., and Fanger, H. (1981) Use of avidin-biotin-peroxidase complex (ABC) in immunoperoxidase techniques. *J. Histochem. Cytochem.* **29,** 577–580.

5. Brigatti, D., Budgeon, L. R., and Unger, E. R. (1988) Immunocytochemistry is automated: Development of a robotic workstation based upon the capillary action principle. *J. Histotechnol.* **11,** 165–170.
6. Yelton, D. E. and Scharff, M. D. (1981) Monoclonal antibodies: A powerful new tool in biology and medicine. *Ann. Rev. Biochem.* **50,** 657–680.
7. Davidoff, M. S. (1986) Immunocytochemistry: Possibilities for detection of different tissue antigens and establishiment of the functional role of cells. *Acta Histochem. Suppl. Band.* **23,** 175–193.
8. Battifora, H. (1991) Assessment of antigen damage in immunohistochemistry. The vimentin internal control. *Am. J. Clin. Pathol.* **96,** 669–671.
9. Reading, M. (1977) A digestion technique for the reducation of background staining in the immunoperoxidase method. *J. Clin. Pathol.* **30,** 88–90.
10. Brozman, M. (1978) Immunohistochemical analyses of formaldehyde and trypsin- or pepsin-treated material. *Acta Histochem.* **63,** 251–260.
11. Heyderman, E. (1979) Immunoperoxidase technique in histopathology: Applications, methods and controls. *J. Clin. Pathol.* **32,** 971–978.
12. Shi, S. R., Key, M. E., and Kalra, K. L. (1991) Antigen retrieval in formalin-fixed paraffin-embedded tissues: An enhancement method for immunohistochemical staining based upon microwave heating of tissue sections. *J. Histochem. Cytochem.* **39,** 741–748.
13. Gown, A. M., de Wever, N., and Battifora, H. (1993) Microwave-based antigenic unmasking. A revolutionary new technique for routine immunohistochemistry. *Appl. Immunohistochem.* **1,** 256–266.
14. Robinson, J. K. (1994) Margin control for lentigo maligna. *J. Am. Acad. Dermatol.* **31,** 79–85.
15. Jimenez, F. J., Grichnik, J. M., Buchanan, M. D., and Clark, R. E. (1995) Immunohistochemical techniques in Mohs micrographic surgery: their potential use in the detection of neoplastic cells masked by inflammation. *J. Am. Acad. Dermatol.* **32,** 89–94.
16. Mondragon, R. M. and Barrett, T. L. (2000) Current concepts: the use of immunoperoxidase techniques in mohs micrographic surgery. *J. Am. Acad. Dermatol.* **43,** 66–71.
17. Nakane, P. K. (1968) Simultaneous localization of multiple tissue antigens using the peroxidase labeled antibody method: A study on pituitary glands of the rat. *J. Histochem. Cytochem.* **16,** 557–560.

II ANTIBODY DIRECTORY

3 Epithelial Markers

Keratins

Pan-Keratin Cocktails

INTRODUCTION

The development of anti-cytokeratin antibodies as diagnostic tools is a long and constantly evolving story. Cytokeratins are one type of intermediate filament that is expressed by epithelial cells. There are currently more than 30 subtypes of cytokeratin. Keratins are divided into two subfamilies based upon isoelectric points *(1)*. Those with pIs less than 5.5 are termed the acidic subfamily and those with pIs greater than 6 are the basic subfamily. Keratinocytes characteristically express pairs of two keratins, one from each subfamily *(2)*. Epithelial cells in different situations express different cytokeratins. For instance, basal keratinocytes normally express cytokeratins 5 and 14. In most circumstances, cytokeratins are expressed with an acidic keratin and a basic keratin produced in tandem. Suprabasilar keratinocytes cease production of these cytokeratins and produce keratins 1 and 10. In conditions of rapid hyperproliferation, the same cells switch over to production of keratins 6 and 16. Cells within hair follicles, eccrine and apocrine glands and nonkeratinizing epithelia in other organ systems produce different keratins. It is largely beyond the scope of a book concerning diagnostic immunopathology to discuss each of the cytokeratin expression patterns. However, it is essential to be aware that anti-cytokeratin cocktails contain mixtures of antibodies directed against only certain subtypes of cytokeratins and that staining results are heavily dependent upon the reagent chosen and the situation examined.

Antibodies directed against specific cytokeratins (such as cytokeratins 5/6, cytokeratin 7 and cytokeratin 20) are described separately.

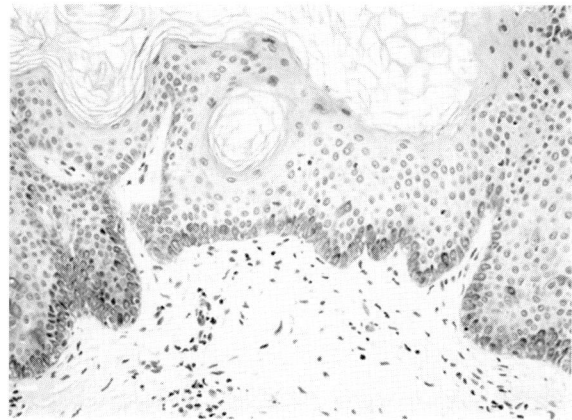

Fig. 1. AE1/AE3 antibodies recognize basal keratinocytes within the epidermis and cutaneous appendages.

Diagnostic Utility

AE1 is a polyclonal cocktail directed against acidic keratins of various molecular weights. It reacts with keratins 10, 14–16, and 19. It recognizes the keratins expressed by normal basal keratinocytes, the secretory cells of eccrine glands, cells in the outer root sheath of hair follicles and the peripheral keratinocytes within sebaceous glands (Fig. 1A,B) *(3)*. It also stains all suprabasilar keratinocytes in situations of hyperproliferation (Fig. 2) *(4)*. It is a useful marker for squamous cell carcinomas, labeling the vast majority of them *(5)*. Entirely spindle shaped, or sarcomatoid squamous cell carcinomas may fail to stain with most anti-keratin markers, including AE1 (Fig. 3) *(6,7)*. AE1 is only weakly and sporadically positive in basal cell carcinomas (mainly in areas with squamous or follicular differentiation) *(5)*. While the antibody recognizes keratins ordinarily expressed by basal keratinocytes (50-kD-keratin) *(8)*, technical problems preclude sensitive labeling in many cases with formalin-fixed, paraffin-embedded tissue.

AE3, another polyclonal antibody that recognizes keratins with molecular weights of 58 kD and 65-67 kD, is expressed by virtually all epidermal cells *(8)*. While it is a good marker for terminal differentiation and keratinization, its lack of further specificity limits its clinical utility. One widely available antibody cocktail combines AE1 and AE3 as a broad-spectrum anti-keratin screen.

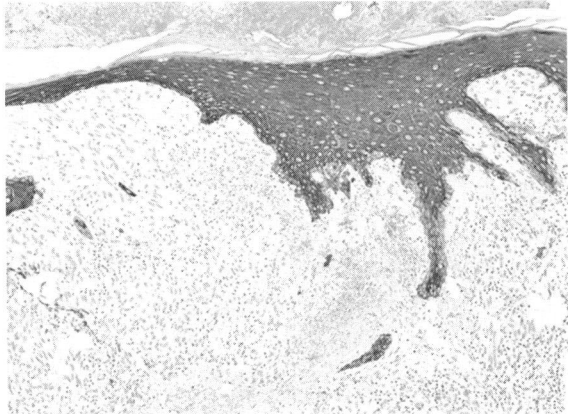

Fig. 2. Suprabasilar staining of keratinocytes with AE1/AE3 in hyper-proliferative states.

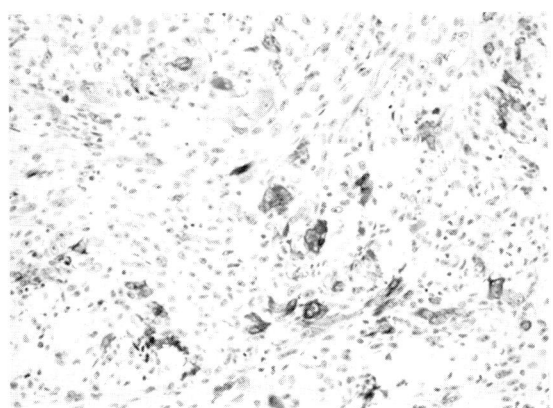

Fig. 3. Spindle cell squamous cell carcinomas often fail to stain with AE1/AE3 antibodies. In this case, only very focal staining was detected.

CAM5.2, another commercially available cocktail directed against a pool of cytokeratins with molecular weights 39 kD, 43 kD, and 50 kD is a good marker for tumors with eccrine differentiation. It is known to react with keratin 18, and perhaps also keratins 8 and 19. It also stains 73% of sebaceous carcinoma *(9).* It is ordinarily not expressed by the keratinocytes in squamous cell carcinomas. About one third of basal cell carcinomas will demonstrate staining with this antibody *(5).* CAM5.2 can be used to identify intraepidermal tumor cells in Paget's disease and extramammary Paget's disease.

MNF116 is another anti-keratin antibody directed against keratins 5, 6, 8, 17, and 19. It has been shown to label basal keratinocytes quite strongly and is a useful marker to identify virtually all squamous cell carcinomas and basal cell carcinomas *(5)*. While MNF116 is clearly a good marker for identifying these tumors, it does not distinguish between them. As there is little call for immunostaining in identifying basal cell carcinomas except in attempting to distinguish these tumors from histologically similar appendageal tumors, all of which label with MNF116, there appears to be little use for this antibody in routine diagnostic laboratories.

In general, anti-keratin antibodies are fairly specific for epithelial cells. However, there are rare reports of anomalous cytokeratin expression by nonepithelial cells. Up to 2% of malignant melanomas have been reported to label with anti-keratin antibodies *(10)*. Epithelioid angiosarcomas may also express cytokeratin *(11,12)*. Expression of cytokeratin is also seen in rare leiomyomas and leiomyosarcomas *(13,14)*. Seminomas, large cell lymphomas and plasma cells can also express keratins. Thus, as with all immunoreagents, interpretation is necessary in reviewing all staining patterns.

Technical Considerations

Anti-cytokeratin antibodies are not as straightforward to use as many of the antibodies in the common repertoire. The protein crosslinking part of the tissue fixation process masks these epitopes markedly decreasing the sensitivity of the antibodies. It is therefore imperative that each laboratory develops a panel of several anti-keratin antibodies that provide reliable staining results. AE1/AE3 and CAM5.2, the two most widely used anti-keratin antibodies, ordinarily require enzymatic digestion as a pretreatment condition. In our laboratory, we pretreat with protease. HIER has also been shown to increase staining intensity *(15)*. Even with antigen retrieval pretreatments, basaloid proliferations stain poorly, if at all with these markers *(5)*.

Summary

There are many commercially available antibodies directed against various combinations of specific cytokeratins. It is not feasible or practical for any laboratory to keep all of them working well. Ideally, a laboratory should stock several overlapping anti-keratin antibodies in order to screen poorly differentiated neoplasms looking for epithelial differentiation. In our laboratory, we routinely use AE1/AE3 in order to establish keratinization. We also use CAM5.2 as a tool for identifying metastatic carcinomas, as well as ductular differentiation, and Merkel cell carcinomas (both of which are better demonstrated with antibodies discussed in the Cytokeratin 7 section). We now use anti-cytokeratin 7 antibodies instead of CAM5.2 in order to identify tumor cells in Paget's disease and extramammary Paget's disease (*see* Chapter 7). Due to its lack of specificity, we do not currently use MNF116 in our laboratory.

Cytokeratin 5/6
Introduction

As has been mentioned already, different types of epithelial cells express different cytokeratins. Cytokeratin 5 is normally expressed by basal keratinocytes and is one of the keratins in the AE1/AE3 antibody cocktail (*see* the Diagnostic Utility section). Cytokeratin 6 is expressed by suprabasilar keratinocytes in hyperproliferative states and is similarly contained in the AE1/AE3 antibody cocktail. Recently, specific antibodies directed against these two specific keratins have been developed.

Diagnostic Utility

The majority of spindle cell squamous cell carcinomas express cytokeratin 5/6 (*16*). This is important in that the previously available cytokeratin antibody cocktails often failed to label spindle cell squamous cell carcinomas. Thus, this new antibody preparation could be very helpful in the immunohistochemical work-up of a spindle cell neoplasm in the skin.

Approximately 10% of epithelioid sarcomas express cytokeratins 5/6 (*17*).

Technical Considerations

Anti-cytokeratin 5/6 antibodies work well on formalin-fixed, paraffin-embedded tissue. It is not yet fully understood exactly why this antibody is able to identify cytokeratins within spindle cells within squamous cell carcinomas that are not recognized by the AE1/AE3 anti-keratin cocktails. Clearly these antibodies are recognizing different epitopes on the cytokeratin 5 and 6 antigens than those targeted by the AE1/AE3 cocktail.

Summary

As this antibody is relatively new, its actual specificities and sensitivities have not been fully elucidated. Thus, as with any new laboratory test, interpretation of results must be performed with caution.

Cytokeratin 7

Introduction

Over the past decade or so, investigators have succeeded in developing stable antibodies directed against many specific cytokeratins. One of the most useful has been the anti-cytokeratin 7 antibody. While cytokeratin 7 is not expressed in normal adult keratinocytes, it is normally expressed on Toker cells and Merkel cells within the epidermis *(18)*.

Diagnostic Utility

Anti-cytokeratin 7 antibodies have a limited, but extremely useful role in diagnostic dermatopathology. The most common situation in which they are employed is in the work-up of mammary or extra-mammary Paget's disease (Fig. 4). It has been demonstrated that cytokeratin 7 is almost always expressed by Paget's cells in either situation, while rarely expressed by the malignant cells in squamous cell carcinomas (Table 1) *(18,19)*. As is unfortunately the case with virtually all antibodies however, the specificity in making this distinction is not 100%. Rare cases of squamous cell carcinoma *in situ* may express cytokeratin 7 *(20)*.

Another common use for anti-cytokeratin 7 antibodies is in the identification of the primary neoplasm in situations with cutaneous metastases from an unknown primary site (Fig. 5). Cytokeratin 7 is known to be expressed on many carcinomas and to be absent from others *(21–24)*. A partial list of extracutaneous neoplasms that express cytokeratin 7 is seen in Table 1.

Cytokeratin 7 is expressed by 23% of Merkel cell carcinomas. While this staining pattern can be helpful in confirming this diagnosis, other antibodies such as cytokeratin 20 are far more sensitive and thus, preferable for this purpose (*see* Chapter 7) *(25)*.

Technical Considerations

Anti-cytokeratin 7 antibodies perform well in routine laboratory conditions. They recognize an epitope that survives formalin fixation

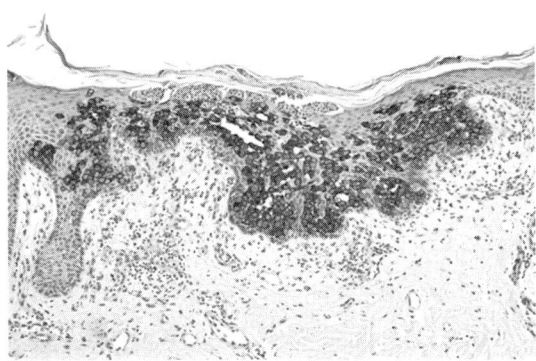

Fig. 4. Intra-epidermal neoplastic cells of Paget's disease strongly express cytokeratin 7.

Table 1
Essentials of Anti-Cytokeratin 7 Antibodies*

	Sensitivity
Paget's disease	95–100%
Extramammary Paget's disease	86%
Other tumors known to express cytokeratin 7	
Urinary bladder	100%
Pancreatic adenocarcinoma	100%
Lung adenocarcinoma	79%
Breast carcinoma	71%
Mesothelioma	67%
Merkel cell carcinoma	23%
Thyroid neoplasms	
Ampullary adenocarcinoma	

*Work on paraffin-embedded, formalin-fixed tissue. Pretreatment not ordinarily required.

and paraffin embedding. Pretreatment is ordinarily necessary in order to maximize staining performance. In our laboratory, we incubate sections with protease prior to the immunostaining procedures.

Summary

Anti-cytokeratin 7 antibodies are useful diagnostic tools for establishing the diagnosis of mammary and extra-mammary Paget's disease. Characterization of adenocarcinomas metastatic to the skin can also be enhanced with use of these antibodies.

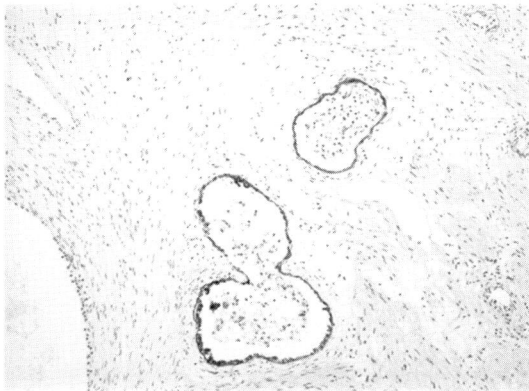

Fig. 5. Glandular epithelium strongly expresses cytokeratin 7.

Cytokeratin 20 (*see* Chapter 7)

Carcinoembryonic Antigen

Introduction

Carcinoembryonic antigen (CEA) is an oncofetal protein that is detected in a wide range of carcinomas (Table 2) *(26)*. The antigen is a protein with a molecular weight of approx 180 kD that is predominantly membranous *(27)*. CEA is found in the developing fetal eccrine glands. This is seen initially as CEA positivity in a single cell within the developing epidermis that evolves into a CEA-positive eccrine unit *(28)*. Within the normal skin, it is routinely present in eccrine and apocrine ducts and glands *(29–31)*. Antibodies to CEA strongly stain the cuticles in these structures *(31)*.

CEA is also believed to be involved in cellular adhesion and may play a role in the development of metastases and in some cutaneous inflammatory processes *(32)*. Anti- CEA is one of the earlier antibodies that became widely available with the development of immunoperoxidase technology. Thus, there is extensive experience with this marker.

Diagnostic Utility

One of the major uses for anti-CEA antibodies is to detect glandular differentiation in cutaneous neoplasms. It is a sensitive marker for Paget's cells. In one study, 100% of cases of extramammary Paget's disease expressed CEA, while only 35% of mammary Paget's dis-

Table 2
Essentials of Anti-Carcinoembryonic Antigen Antibodies*

Tumors known to express CEA	Sensitivity
Extramammary Paget's disease	100%
Paget's disease	35–100%
Cutaneous lymphadenoma	
Stomach adenocarcinoma	
Colonic adenocarcinoma	
Pancreatic adenocarcinoma	
Lung adenocarcinoma	
Cervical adenocarcinoma	

*Work well on paraffin-embedded, formalin-fixed tissue. Polyclonal and monoclonal antibodies available.

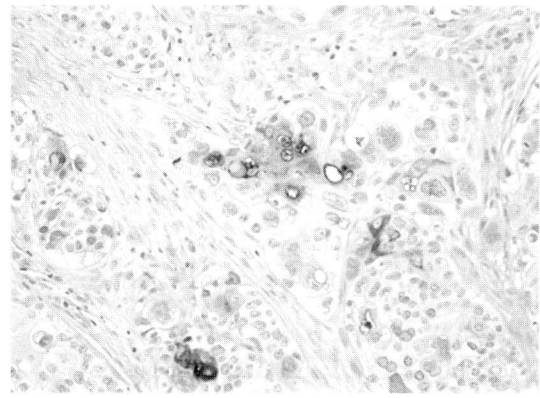

Fig. 6. Ductular lining cells in eccrine neoplasms express CEA.

ease cases were positive with this antibody *(29)*. However, others have detected CEA in a higher percentage of cases of mammary Paget's disease *(33)*. Other studies have confirmed the relatively high specificity for anti-CEA antibodies in the differential diagnosis of intraepidermal Pagetoid cells *(34)*.

Anti-CEA is a relatively sensitive marker for benign and malignant eccrine and apocrine neoplasms (Fig. 6) *(35)*. It stains up to 75% of both benign and malignant eccrine tumors *(36)*. Sebaceous carcinomas show staining with anti-CEA antibodies in sebocytes, ducts and cysts, and in keratotic foci *(37)*. CEA positivity within cutaneous lymphadenomas supports the notion that these represent cutaneous adnexal neoplasms *(38)*.

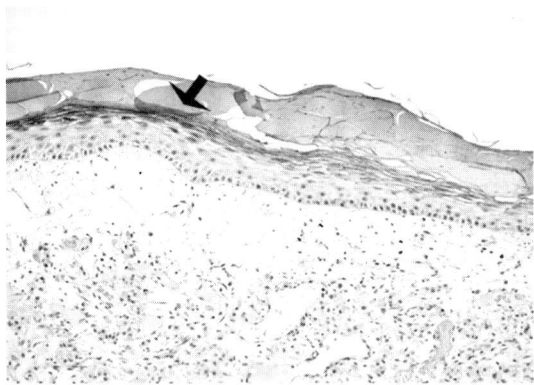

Fig. 7. The stratum corneum nonspecifically stains with anti-CEA antibodies in many cases.

In some inflammatory conditions, CEA expression can be detected in keratinocytes in the upper layers of the epidermis *(32)*. CEA is not ordinarily expressed by basal keratinocytes, nor by basal cell carcinomas; however, in a subset of such carcinomas arising in black patients, CEA expression has been detected *(39)*. It is also seen in basal cell carcinomas that display sebaceous differentiation *(37)*.

CEA expression is detected by the majority of cutaneous melanomas using a polyclonal anti-CEA antibody, but is not ordinarily found with monoclonal anti-CEA antibodies. A similar reaction pattern is seen in cutaneous deposits of metastatic melanoma *(27)*. It has subsequently been demonstrated that melanomas express the sialyl Lewis x carbohydrate moiety of CEA, but do not actually express CEA itself *(40)*. Polyclonal antibodies to CEA label up to 80% of squamous cell carcinomas *(41)*.

Technical Considerations

CEA antibodies tend to stain with a high background (Fig. 7). These antibodies are easy to use and work quite well in formalin-fixed, paraffin-embedded tissue sections. Enzymatic or HIER pretreatment is usually necessary to maximize performance *(15)*. However, they almost always diffusely stain the entire stratum corneum, giving a high background blush to stained sections. In most cases, this staining does not preclude interpretation, but in many cases, higher signal to noise ratios can be attained with other antibodies to reveal similar information.

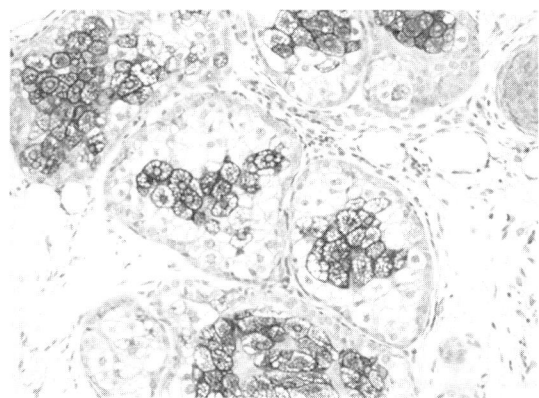

Fig. 8. Mature sebocytes express EMA, but the basaloid cells at the periphery of sebaceous glands do not.

Summary

Anti-CEA is a good general screening reagent. It is useful for providing support for glandular differentiation in primary skin tumors or in tumors metastatic to the skin. It is also useful in establishing a diagnosis of mammary or extra-mammary Paget's disease. In my experience, however, it is a relatively "dirty" antibody to interpret and is expressed by such a wide range of neoplasms as to be relatively nonspecific. While I keep this antibody in the laboratory, I use it only to provide additional support for diagnoses establishing based upon the staining pattern of other antibodies.

Epithelial Membrane Antigen (EMA)

Introduction

Epithelial membrane antigen (EMA) characteristically is expressed on the apical and luminal surfaces of some glandular epithelial cells *(42,43)*. An antibody raised against human fat globule membranes recognizes this protein *(44)*. It is not ordinarily expressed on normal adult skin, but it is present on normal fetal epidermis prior to keratinization *(45)*. EMA is usually present on the luminal surfaces and lateral borders of both apocrine and eccrine glands, but is not present within the ducts *(46)*. Perineurial cells also express EMA *(47)*. Mature sebocytes express EMA but the antigen is not ordinarily expressed by immature sebocytes (Fig. 8) *(48)*.

Table 3
Essentials of Anti-Epithelial Membrane Antigen Antibodies*

Neoplasms known to express EMA	Sensitivity
Squamous cell carcinoma	100%
Small cell anaplastic carcinoma	100%
Mesothelioma	100%
Adenocarcinoma	91%
Breast	
Colon	
Lung	
Stomach	
Pancreas	
Gallbladder	
Prostate	
Ovary	
Kidney	
Thyroid	
Leiomyosarcoma	44%
Chordoma	25%
Melanoma	6.5%
Synovial sarcoma	
Epithelioid sarcoma	
Myoepithelioma	

*Monoclonal antibody, work well in paraffin-embedded, formalin-fixed tissue, and do not ordinarily require pretreatment.

Diagnostic Utility

Anti-EMA is a very useful antibody in diagnostic dermatopathology. The antibody suffers from a lack of absolute specificity and sensitivity, but nonetheless can be very helpful in certain situations and when used in conjunction with other, more specific and sensitive markers. EMA is expressed by many tumors, some of which are listed in Table 3. EMA is also expressed by some hematopoietic cells, including plasma cells, Reed Sternberg cells, and the neoplastic lymphocytes in large cell anaplastic lymphomas (42,49–51). Myoepithelial cells in myoepitheliomas are known to express EMA (52).

Labeling with anti-EMA antibodies is helpful in determining eccrine differentiation in cutaneous neoplasms (Fig. 9). Hidradenomas, poromas and syringomas almost always express EMA (46,53,54). Similarly, sebaceous carcinomas are usually strongly positive with anti-EMA antibody (55). Microvesiculation within

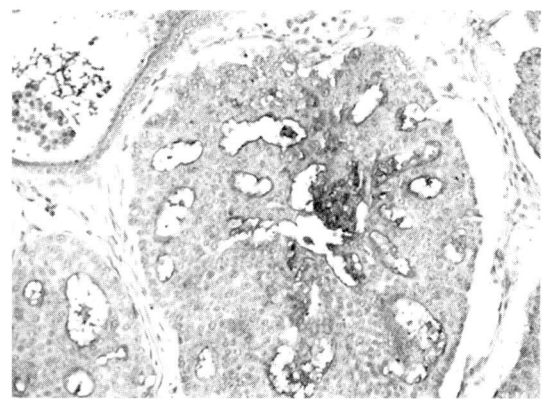

Fig. 9. Ductular lining cells in eccrine and apocrine neoplasms label with anti-EMA antibodies.

mature sebocytes is clearly outlined by this antibody. This can be a helpful diagnostic feature. Squamous cell carcinomas, both invasive and *in situ*, usually express EMA with a focal, patchy pattern *(37,45)*. The cells in both mammary and extramammary Paget's disease strongly express EMA in the vast majority of cases *(56)*.

Some unexpected neoplasms may also express EMA. Rare melanomas have been reported to stain with anti-EMA. The staining is usually quite faint *(57)*. Leiomyosarcomas express EMA in almost 50% of cases *(58)*.

Identification of EMA expression is helpful in making a diagnosis of cutaneous lymphadenoma and lymphoepithelioma, and has also provided insight into the pathogenesis of these uncommon neoplasms *(59,60)*. Neurothekeomas and perineuromas can be identified with the help of EMA localization to the perineurium *(47)*.

Technical Considerations

Monoclonal anti-EMA antibodies are easy to use and work well in formalin-fixed, paraffin-embedded tissue sections. They provide a very clean staining pattern with excellent, low levels of background staining. Pretreatment with enzymes or microwave antigen retrieval is ordinarily not required but has been shown to increase signal intensity *(15)*.

Summary

Anti-EMA is a valuable reagent in a diagnostic dermatopathology laboratory. It can used as a first line tool in screening for glandular differentiation, establishing or confirming a diagnosis of Paget's disease (or extramammary Paget's disease), or even providing additional support for a diagnosis of large cell lymphoma. It is probably not a good choice as a single reagent for any of these purposes. Nonetheless, it has a broad enough spectrum of uses to be a cost-effective reagent for general laboratory usage.

Gross Cystic Disease Fluid Protein
Introduction

Gross cystic disease fluid protein (GCDFP-15) is a major proteinaceous component of breast cysts. It has been detected in normal glandular epithelium in the skin, salivary gland, bronchial glands, prostate, seminal vesicles, and breast tissue *(61)*.

Diagnostic Utility

Anti- GCDFP-15 stains the cells in Paget's and extramammary Paget's disease *(62)*. In extramammary Paget's disease, GCDFP-15 expression has been associated with primary cutaneous lesions that have no underlying associated malignancy. The absence of such staining within these Pagetoid cells is associated with underlying gastrointestinal or genitourinary neoplasms *(62,63)*.

Anti-GCDFP-15 has been shown to stain close to 100% of primary cutaneous apocrine neoplasms *(64)*. A similar percentage of benign and malignant eccrine neoplasms will express GCDFP-15 *(65)*.

GCDFP-15 expression is also helpful in identifying cutaneous metastases as being of potential breast origin. However, as primary cutaneous eccrine and apocrine neoplasms can also express this protein, identification of GCDFP-15 expression does not distinguish metastatic breast carcinoma from primary cutaneous glandular neoplasms *(66,67)*. (There is not yet a reproducible method for making this distinction using immunopathology.) GCDFP-15 expression has not been detected in metastatic neoplasms from other primary sites.

Technical Considerations

GCDFP-15 is a widely available antibody that works well on routinely processed tissue sections. While enzymatic or heat-induced epitope retrieval is not essential, both have been shown to increase staining intensity *(15)*.

Summary

Anti-GCDFP-15 is a useful confirmatory antibody for the diagnostic dermatopathology laboratory. The range of neoplasms identified by the antibody is relatively limited and is largely duplicated by antibodies such as anti-cytokeratin 7, anti-EMA, and anti-CEA. Thus, anti-GCDFP-15 is not an essential reagent for a laboratory. Whether or not to stock it is largely a matter of preference in working with this or several of the other markers useful for detecting cutaneous appendageal neoplasms. We do not currently use this antibody in our laboratory.

Sex–Hormone Receptors

Introduction

The skin in certain anatomic locations may express various sex hormone receptors. Androgen receptors are present in keratinocytes, sebaceous glands, eccrine glands, follicular epithelium, and dermal fibroblasts within vaginal skin *(68)*. Estrogen receptors are present in vaginal mucosal epithelium and in the basal keratinocytes of vulvar skin. They are also present in stromal fibroblasts, and smooth muscle cells in these locations. Vaginal epithelial cells, fibroblasts and smooth muscle cells express progesterone receptors, while cells in vulvar skin do not *(68)*. While not so clearly demarcated, expression of these receptors has been reported in other cutaneous locations. Specifically, sebaceous glands are almost always positive with antibodies directed against these proteins, as are many eccrine and apocrine gland cells. Follicular keratinocytes demonstrate variable expression depending upon growth phases *(69)*.

Diagnostic Utility

There are relatively limited diagnostic uses in dermatopathology for antibodies directed against estrogen receptors, progesterone receptors and androgen receptors. These antibodies can be helpful in identifying carcinomas metastatic to the skin, most often breast carcinomas (Fig. 10) *(70)*. However, as there is some overlap in the sensitivity and specificity, positive staining with any of these antibodies cannot be used to absolutely distinguish metastatic breast carcinoma from primary cutaneous eccrine neoplasm *(66,71,72)*. In a large study, 21% of sweat gland carcinomas and 33% of breast

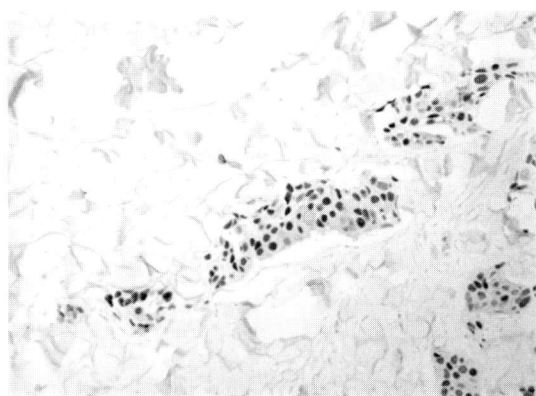

Fig. 10. Antibodies directed against estrogen receptors display strong nuclear staining in this case of breast carcinoma metastatic to the skin.

carcinomas metastatic to the skin expressed estrogen receptors. Similarly, 19% of sweat gland carcinomas expressed progesterone receptors, as did 27% of metastatic breast carcinomas *(73)*.

Androgen receptors can be found in some cases of extramammary Paget's disease, but estrogen and progesterone receptors are almost always absent *(74)*.

Early studies suggested the possibility that melanomas, congenital nevi and dysplastic nevi expressed estrogen and progesterone receptors, unlike ordinary acquired nevi *(75–78)*. However, this finding has not been attained in a reproducible manner, and is not thought to be a reliable diagnostic discriminator.

Technical Considerations

Commercially available antibodies directed against epitopes of estrogen receptors, progesterone receptors and androgen receptors that survive routine processing are readily available. These antibodies require enzymatic pretreatment or HIER in order to perform well in formalin-fixed, paraffin-embedded tissue sections *(15)*. High background staining may be a problem, especially for anti-progesterone antibody stained sections.

Summary

While antibodies directed against estrogen receptors, progesterone receptors and androgen receptors might be helpful in confirming a diagnosis of breast carcinoma metastatic to the skin, they are not 100% sensitive or specific for this diagnosis. Other markers may be equally useful in making this diagnosis and serve other diagnostic functions. These antibodies may prove to be useful in determining pathogeneses of various cutaneous conditions, but at this point have only a limited role in diagnostic dermatopathology.

References

1. Smack, D. P., Korge, B. P., and James, W. D. (1994) Keratin and keratinization. *J. Am. Acad. Dermatol.* **30,** 85–102.
2. Eichner, R., Bonitz, P., and Sun, T. T. (1984) Classification of epidermal keratins according to their immunoreactivity, isoelectric point, and mode of expression. *J. Cell Biol.* **98,** 1388–1396.
3. Ansai, S. I., Katagata, Y., Yoshikawa, K. I., Hozumi, Y., and Aso, K. (1993) Keratin specificity analyses of eight anti-keratin monoclonal antibodies, and their immunostaining pattersn in normal skin using formalin-fixed and paraffin-embedded tissue specimens. *Arch. Dermatol. Res.* **285,** 6–12.
4. Weiss, R. A., Eichner, R., and Sun, T. T. (1984) Monoclonal antibody analysis of keratin expression in epidermal diseases: a 48- and 56- kdalton keratin as molecular markers for hyperproliferative keratinocytes. *J. Cell Biol.* **98,** 1397–1406.
5. Prieto, V. G., Lugo, J., and McNutt, N. S. (1996) Intermediate- and low-molecular weight keratin detection with the monoclonal antibody MNF116. An immunohistochemical study on 232 paraffin-embedded cutaneous lesions. *J Cutan. Pathol.* **23,** 234–241.
6. Avagnina, A., Juarez, M. A., and Elsner, B. (1990) Spindle cell carcinomas. Immunohistochemical analysis of 15 cases. *Medicina (B Aires)* **50,** 325–329.
7. Gray, Y., Robidoux, H. J., Farrell, D. S., and Robinson-Bostom, L. (2001) Squamous cell carcinoma detected by high-molecular-weight cytokeratin immunostaining mimicking atypical fibroxanthoma. *Arch. Pathol. Lab. Med.* **125,** 799–802.
8. Woodcock-Mitchell, J., Eichner, R., Nelson, W. G., and Sun, T. T. (1982) Immunolocalization of keratin polypeptides in human epidermis using monoclonal antibodies. *J. Cell. Biol.* **95,** 580–588.
9. Murata, T., Nakashima, Y., Takeuchi, M., Sueshi, K., and Inomata, H. (1993) the diagnostic use of low molecular weight keratin expression in sebaceous carcinoma. *Pathol. Res. Pract.* **189,** 888–893.
10. Zarbo, R. J., Gown, A. M., Nagle, R. B., Visscher, D., and Crissman, J. D. (1990) Anomalous cytokeratin expression in malignant melanoma: one- and two-dimensional western blot analysis and immunohistochemical survey of 100 melanomas. *Mod. Pathol.* **3,** 494–501.
11. Smith, K. J., Lupton, G. P., and Skelton, H. G., III (1997) Cutaneous angiosarcomas with a starry-sky pattern. *Arch. Pathol. Lab. Med.* **121,** 980–984.
12. McCluggage, W. G., Clarke, R., and Toner, P.G. (1995) Cutaneous epithelioid angiosarcoma exhibiting cytokeraitn positivity. *Histopathology* **27,** 291–294.
13. Kaddu, S., Beham, A., Cerroni, L., Humer-Fuchs, U., Salmhofer, W., Kerl, H., and Soyer, H. P. (1997) Cutaneous leiomyosarcoma. *Am. J. Surg. Pathol.* **21,** 979–987.

14. Lundgren, L., Kindblom, L. G., Seidal, T., and Angervall, L. (1991) Intermediate and fine cytofilaments in cutaneous and subcutaneous leiomyosarcomas. *APMIS* **99**, 820–828.

15. Gown, A. M., de Wever, N., and Battifora, H. (1993) Microwave-based antigenic unmasking. A revolutionary new technique for routine immunohistochemistry. *Appl. Immunohistochem.* **1**, 256–266.

16. Sigel, J. E., Skacel, M., Bergfeld, W. F., House, N. S., Rabkin, M. S., and Goldblum, J.R. (2001) The utility of cytokeratin 5/6 in the recognition of cutaneous spindle cell squamous cell carcinoma. *J. Cutan. Pathol.* **28**, 520–524.

17. Lin, L., Sigel, J. E., Bergfeld, W. F., and Goldblum, J. R. (2001) Epithelioid sarcoma: an immunohistochemical analysis of cytokeratin 5/6 and cyclin D1 (abstract). *J. Cutan. Pathol.* **28**, 574.

18. Lundquist, K., Kohler, S., and Rouse, S. V. (1999) Intraepidermal cytokeratin 7 expression is not restricted to paget cells, but is also seen in Toker cells and Merkel cells. *Am. J. Surg. Pathol.* **23**, 212–219.

19. Brainard, J. A. and Hart, W. R. (2000), Proliferative epidermal lesions associated with anogenital Paget's disease. *Am. J. Surg. Pathol.* **24**, 543–552.

20. Williamson, J. D., Colome, M. I., Sahin, A., Ayala, A. G., and Medeiros, L. J. (2000) Pagetoid bowen disease: a report of 2 cases that express cytokeratin 7. *Arch. Pathol. Lab. Med.* **124**, 427–430.

21. Chu, P., Wu, E., and Weiss, L. M. (2000) Cytokeratin 7 and cytokeratin 20 expression in epithelial neoplasms: a survey of 435 cases. *Mod. Pathol.* **13**, 962–972.

22. Jiang, J., Ulbright, T. M., Younger, C., Sanchez, K., Bostwick, D. G., Koch, M. O., et al. (2001) Cytokeratin 7 ad cytokeratin 20 in primary urinary bladder carcinoma and matched lymph node metastases. *Arch. Pathol. Lab. Med.* **125**, 921–923.

23. Fernandez, C., Liprandi, A., Bouvier-Labit, C., and Figarella-Branger, D. (2001) Value of cytokeratin 7 and 20 for the diagnosis of cerebral metastases of adenocarcinoma: study of 78 cases. *Ann. Pathol.* **21**, 129–135.

24. Goldstein, N.S. and Bassi, D. (2001) Cytokeratins 7, 17, and 20 reactivity in pancreatic and ampulla of Vater adenocarcinomas. Percentage of positivity and distribution is affected by the cut-point threshold. *Am. J. Clin. Pathol.* **115**, 695–702.

25. Jensen, K., Kohler, S., and Rouse, R. V. (2000) cytokeratin staining in Merkel cell carcinoma: an immunohistochemical study of cytokeratins 5/6, 7, 17, and 20. *Appl. Immunohistochem. Molecul. Morphol.* **8**, 310–315.

26. Goldenberg, D. M., Sharkey, R. M., and Primus, F. J., (1976) Carcinoembryonic antigen in histopathology: immunoperoxidase staining of conventional tissue sections. *J. Natl. Cancer Inst.* **57**, 11–22.

27. Sanders, D. S., Evans, A. T., Allen, C. A., Bryant, F. J., Johnson, G. D., Hopkins, J., et al. (1994) Classification of CEA-related positivity in primary and metastatic malignant melanoma. *J. Pathol.* **172**, 343–348.

28. Penneys, N. S., Kott-Blumenkrantz, R., and Buck, B. E. (1984) Carcinoembryonic antigen in fetal eccrine glands: an immunohistochemical study. *Pediatr. Dermatol.* **1**, 281–282.

29. Guarner, J., Cohen, C., and DeRose, P. B. (1989), Histogenesis of extramammary and mammary Paget's cells. an immunohistochemical study. *Am. J. Dermatopathol.* **11**, 313–318.

30. Inaba, Y., Egawa, K., Kageshita, T., and Ono, T. (1992) Expression of CA 50 in normal human skin: comparative study of CEA and CA 19–9. *J. Dermatol.* **19**, 592–597.

31. Penneys, N. S., Nadji, M., and McKinney, E. C. (1981) Carcinoembryonic antigen present in human eccrine sweat. *J. Am. Acad. Dermatol.* **4**, 401–403.

32. Egawa, K., Honda, Y., Kuroki, M., Inaba, Y., and Ono, T. (1996) Carcino-embryonic antigen and related antigens expressed on keratinocytes in inflammatory dermatoses. *Brit. J. Dermatol.* **134,** 451–459.

33. Nadji, M., Morales, A. R., Girtanner, R. E., Ziegels-Weissman, J., and Penneys, N. S. (1982) Paget's disease of the skin. A unifying concept of histogenesis. *Cancer* **50,** 2203–2206.

34. Guldhammer, B. and Norgard, T. (1986) The differential diagnosis of intraepidermal malignant lesions using immunohistochemistry. *Am. J. Dermatopathol.* **8,** 295–301.

35. Penneys, N. S., Nadji, M., Zeigels-Weissman, J., Ketabchi, M., and Morales, A. R. (1982), Carcinoembryonic antigen in sweat-gland carcinomas. *Cancer* **50,** 1608–1611.

36. Mairoana, A., Nigrisoli, E., and Papotti, M. (1986) Immunohistochemical markers of sweat gland tumors. *J. Cutan. Pathol.* **13,** 187–196.

37. Heyderman, E., Graham, R. M., Chapman, D. V., Richardson, T. C., and McKee, P. H. (1984) Epithelial markers in primary skin cancer: an immunoperoxidase study of the distribution of epithelial membrane antigen (EMA) and carcino-embryonic antigen (CEA) in 65 primary skin carcinomas. *Histopathology* **8,** 423–434.

38. Requena, L. and Sanchez Yus, E. (1992) Cutaneous lymphadenoma with ductal differentiation. *J. Cutan. Pathol.* **19,** 429–433.

39. Carcinoembryonic antigen in basal cell neoplasms in black patients: an immunohistochemical study. *J. Am. Acad. Dermatol.* **21,** 1007–1010.

40. Ravindranath, M. H., Shen, P., Habal, N., Soh, D., Nishimoto, K., Gonzales, A., et al. (2000) Does human melanoma express carcinoembryonic antigen? *Anticancer Res.* **20,** 3083–3092.

41. Ariano, M. C., Wiley, E. L., Ariano, L., Coon, J. S. T., and Tetzlaff, L. (1985) H, peanut lectin receptor, and carcinoembryonic antigen distribution in keratoacanthomas, squamous dysplasias, and carcinomas of the skin. *J. Dermatol. Surg. Oncol.* **11,** 1076–1083.

42. Pinkus, G. S. and Kurtin, P. J. (1985) Epithelial membrane antigen—a diagnostic discriminant in surgical pathology: immunohistochemical profile in epithelial, mesenchymal, and hematopoietic neoplasms using paraffin sections and monoclonal antibodies. *Hum. Pathol.* **16,** 929–940.

43. Petersen, O. W. and cvan Deurs, B. (1986) Characterizatin of epithelial membrane antigen expression in human mammary epithelium by ultrastructural immunoperoxidase cytochemistry. *J. Histochem. Cytochem.* **34,** 801–809.

44. Sloane, J. P. and Ormerod, M. G. (1981) Distribution of epithelial membrane antigen in normal and neoplastic tissues and its value in diagnostic tumor pathology. *Cancer* **47,** 1786–1795.

45. Sloane, J. P., Ormerod, M. G., Carter, R. L., Gusterson, B. A., and Foster, C. S. (1982) An immunocytochemical study of the distribution of epithelial membrane antigen in normal and disordered squamous epithelium. *Diagn. Histopathol.* **5,** 11–17.

46. Noda, Y., Horike, H., Watanabe, Y., Mori, M., and Tsujimura, T. (1987) Immunohistochemical identification of epithelial membrane antigen in sweat gland tumors by the use of a monoclonal antibody. *Pathol. Res. Pract.* **182,** 797–804.

47. Percentes, E., Nakagawa, Y., Ross, G. W., Stanton, C., and Rubinstein, L. J. (1987) Expression of epithelial membrane antigen in perineurial cells and their derivatives. An immunohistochemical study with multiple markers. *Acta Neuropathol. (Berl).* **75,** 160–165.

48. Latham, J. A., Redfern, C. P., Thody, A. J., and De Krester, T. A. (1989) Immunohistochemical markers of human sebaceous gland differentiation. *J. Histochem. Cytochem.* **37,** 729–734.

49. Ross, C. W., Hanson, C. A., and Schnitzer, B. (1992) CD30 (Ki-1)- positive, anaplastic large cell lymphoma mimicking gastarointestinal carcinoma. *Cancer* **70,** 2517–2523.

50. Stein, H., Hansmann, M. L., Lennert, K., Brandtzaeg, P., Gatter, K. C., and Mason, D. Y. (1986) Reed-Sternberg and Hodgkin's cells in lymphocyte-predominant Hodgkin's disease of nodular subtype contain J chain. *Am. J. Clin. Pathol.* **86,** 292–297.

51. Sassser, R. L., Yam, L. T., and Li, C. Y. (1990) Myeloma with involvement of the serous cavities. Cytologic and immunochemical diagnosis and literature review. *Acta Cytol.* **34,** 479–485.

52. Kutzner, H., Mentzel, T., Kaddu, S., Soares, L. M., Sangueza, O. P., and Requena, L. (2001) Cutaneous myoepithelioma: an under-recognized cutaneous neoplasm composed of myoepithelial cells. *Am. J. Surg. Pathol.* **25,** 348–355.

53. Haupt, H. M., Stern, J. B., and Berlin, S. J. (1992) Immunohistochemistry in the differential diagnosis of nodular hidradenoma and glomus tumor. *Am. J. Dermatopathol.* **14,** 310–314.

54. Swanson, P. E., Cherwitz, D. L., Neumann, M. P., and Wick, M. R. (1987) Eccrine sweat gland carcinoma: an histologic and immunohistochemical study of 32 cases. *J. Cutan. Pathol.* **14,** 65–86.

55. Ansai, S., Hashimoto, H., Aoki, T., Hozumi, Y., and Aso, K. (1993) A histochemical and immunohistochemical study of extra-ocular sebaceous carcinoma. *Histopathology* **22,** 127–133.

56. Vanstapel, M. J., Gatter, K. C., De Wolf-Peeters, C., Millard, P. R., Desmet, V. J., and Mason, D. Y. (1984) Immunohistochemical study of mammary and extra-mammary Paget's disease. *Histopathology* **8,** 1013–1023.

57. Ben-Izhak, O., Stark, P., Levy, R., Bergman, R., and Lichtig, C. (1994) Epithelial markers in malignant melanoma. A study of primary lesions and their metastases. *Am. J. Dermatopathol.* **16,** 241–246.

58. Iata, J. and Fletcher, C. D. (2000) Immunohistochemical detection of cytokeratin and epithelial membrane antigen in leiomyosarcoma: a systematic study of 100 cases. *Pathol. Int.* **50,** 7–14.

59. Santa Cruz, D. J., Barr, R. J., and Headington, J. T. (1991) Cutaneous lymphadenoma. *Am. J. Surg. Pathol.* **15,** 101–110.

60. Swanson, S. A., Cooper, P. H., Mills, S. E., and Wick, M. R. (1988) Lymphoepithelioma-like carcinoma of the skin. *Mod. Pathol.* **1,** 359–365.

61. Satoh, F., Umemura, S., and Osamura, R. Y. (2000) Immunohistochemical analysis of CGDFP-15 and GCDFP-24 in mammary and nonmammary tissue. *Breast Cancer* **7,** 49–55.

62. Nowak, M. A., Guerriere-Kovach, P., Pathan, A., Campbell, T. E., and Deppisch, L. M. (1998) Perianal Paget's disease: distinguishing primary and secondary lesions using immunohistochemical studies including gross cystic disease fluid protein-15 and cytokeratin 20 expression. *Arch. Pathol. Lab. Med.* **122,** 1077–1081.

63. Kohler, S. and Smoller, B. R. (1996) Gross cystic disease fluid protein-15 reactivity in extramammary Paget's disease with and without associated internal malignancy. *Am. J. Dermatopathol.* **18,** 118–123.

64. Ansai, S., Koseki, S., Hozumi, Y., and Kondo, S. (1995) An immunohistochemical study of lysozyme, CD-15 (Leu-M1), and gross cystic disease fluid protein-15 in various skin tumors. Assessment of the spcificity and sensitivity of markers of apocrine differentiation. *Am. J. Dermatopathol.* **17,** 249–255.

65. Mazoujian, G. and Margolis, R. (1988) Immunohistochemistry of gross cystic disease fluid protein (GCDFP-15) in 65 benign sweat gland tumors of the skin. *Am. J. Dermatopathol.* **10,** 28–35.

66. Wallace, M. L., Longacre, T. A., and Smoller, B. R. (1995) Estrogen and progresterone receptors and anti-gross cystic disease fluid protein 15 (BRST-2) fail to distinguish metastatic breast carcinoma from eccrine neoplasms. *Mod. Pathol.* **8,** 897–901.

67. Ormsby, A. H., Snow, J. L., Su, W. P., and Goellner, J. R. (1995) Diagnostic immunohistochemistry of cutaneous metastatic breast carcinoma: a statistical analysis of the utility of gross cystic disease fluid protein-15 and estrogen receptor protein. *J. Am. Acad. Dermatol.* **32,** 711–716.

68. Hodgins, M. B., Spike, R. C., Mackie, R. M., and MacLean, A. B. (1998) An immunohistochemical study of androgen, oestrogen and progesterone receptors in the vulva and vagina. *Brit. J. Obstet. Gynaecol.* **105,** 216–222.

69. Wallace, M. L. and Smoller, B. R. (1998) Estrogen and progesterone receptors in androgenic alopecia versus alopecia areata. *Am. J. Dermatopathol.* **20,** 160–163.

70. Wallace, M. L. and Smoller, B. R. (1996) Differential sensitivity of estrogen/progesterone receptors and BRST-2 markers in metastatic ductal and lobular breast carcinoma to the skin. *Am. J. Dermatopathol.* **18,** 241–247.

71. Carson, H. J., Gattuso, P., Raslan, W. F., and Reddy, V. B. (1995) Mucinous carcinoma of the eyelid. An immunohistochemical study. *Am. J. Dermatopathol.* **17,** 484–498.

72. Wick, M. R., Ockner, D. M., Mills, S. E., Ritter, J. H., and Swanson, P. E. (1998) Homologus carcinomas of the breasts, skin, and salivary glands. A histologic and immunohistochemical comparison of ductal mammary carcinoma, ductal sweat carcinoma, and salivary duct carcinoma. *Am. J. Clin. Pathol.* **109,** 75–84.

73. Busam, K. J., Tan, L. K., Granter, S. R., Kohler, S., Junkins-Hopkins, J., Berwick, M., and Rosen, P. P. (1999) Epidermal growth factor, estrogen, and progesterone receptor expression in primary sweat gland carcinomas and primary and metastatic mammary carcinomas. *Mod. Pathol.* **12,** 786–793.

74. Diaz de Leon, E., Carcangui, M. L., Prieto, V. G., McCue, P. A., Burchette, J. L., To, G., et al. (2000) Extramammary Paget's disease is characterized by the consistent lack of estrogen and progesterone receptors but frequently expresses androgen receptor. *Am. J. Clin. Pathol.* **113,** 572–575.

75. Thompson, A. J., Cook, M. G., and Gill, P. G. (1981) Immunofluorescent detection of hormone receptors in cutaneous melanocytic tumores. *Brit. J. Cancer* **43,** 644–653.

76. Sawaya, M. E., Garland, L. D., Rothe, M. J., Honig, L. S., and Hsia, S. L. (1988) Oestrogen and progesterone receptors in lentigo maligna. *Brit. J. Dermatol.* **118,** 69–71.

77. Ellis, D. L., Wheeland, R. G., and Solomon, H. (1985) Estrogen and progesterone receptors in congenital melanocytic nevi. *J. Am. Acad. Dermatol.* **12,** 235–244.

78. Ellis, D. L., Wheeland, R. G., and Solomon, H. (1985) Estrogen and progesterone receptors in primary cutaneous melanoma. *J. Dermatol. Surg. Oncol.* **11,** 54–59.

4 Mesenchymal Markers (Nonhematopoietic)

Vimentin

Introduction

Vimentin is one of the types of intermediate (10 nm) filaments that characterize cell types. It is a 57 kD protein and is expressed primarily in cells of mesenchymal origin. Immunogold labeling localized vimentin to the cytoplasmic processes of fibroblasts, Langerhans cells and melanocytes, with lesser amounts in the peri-nuclear cytoplasm *(1)*. Anti-vimentin antibodies were among the first antibodies available for diagnostic use. Early studies suggested that vimentin expression was relatively specific and that its detection in cells would enable diagnosticians to categorize a tumor as being of mesenchymal origin *(2,3)*. Almost immediately thereafter, it was discovered that vimentin could be detected in cells that were nonmesenchymal. Normal and malignant melanocytes (of neuroectodermal origin) were found to strongly express vimentin *(4–6)*. Within several years, the list of neoplasms known to express vimentin had grown significantly, and thus, its diagnostic specificity became less impressive *(7)*.

Diagnostic Utility

As vimentin expression has been detected in an ever-expanding number of neoplasms, its diagnostic utility has progressively lessened. In distinguishing between undifferentiated carcinomas and melanomas, strong vimentin expression may favor melanoma. However, this distinction is made much more easily and directly with use of the relatively melanocyte-specific markers such as MART-1, HMB-45 or tyrosinase (*see* Chapter 6).

In the more subtle distinction of spindle cell neoplasms in the skin, vimentin is similarly limited. All mesenchymally derived neoplasms such as leiomyosarcomas, dermatofibrosarcoma protuberans, glomus tumors, and atypical fibroxanthomas express vimentin (Fig. 1) *(8,9)*. Further, endothelial cell derived tumors (also mesenchymal) express this protein. Thus, vimentin expression does nothing to dis-

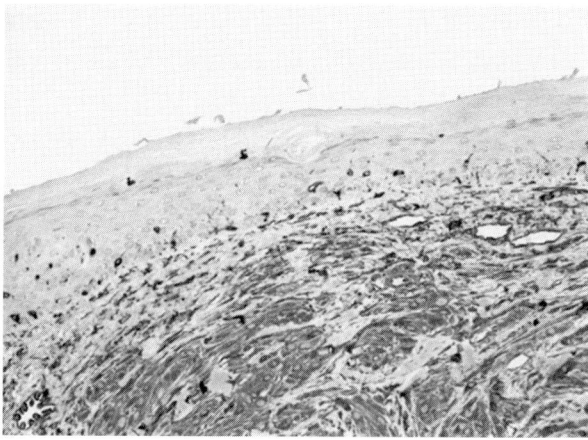

Fig. 1. Vimentin is expressed strongly by most mesenchymally derived neoplasms. Note also the strong staining of Langerhans cells and melanocytes within the epidermis by anti-vimentin antibodies.

criminate between these neoplasms. Further exacerbating the problem is the relatively newer finding that squamous cell carcinomas with a spindle-shaped morphology can be expected to express vimentin, as can spindle cell melanomas *(10,11)*. In one series, 40% of spindle cell squamous cell carcinomas expressed vimentin *(12)*. Thus, virtually every neoplasm occurring within the skin that may demonstrate a spindle cell morphology would likely be detected by anti-vimentin antibodies.

Rare cutaneous neoplasms with a more epithelial morphology, such as lymphoepithelioma-like carcinomas, lymphadenomas and rhabdoid tumors may also display vimentin filaments in the epithelial components *(13–15)*.

In the work-up of metastatic neoplasms involving the skin, vimentin positivity must be interpreted with caution, as renal cell carcinomas, endometrial adenocarcinomas, thyroid carcinomas, adrenocortical adenomas, adenocarcinomas of the lungs, ovaries, salivary glands, prostate, and breast have all been shown to express vimentin *(12)*.

Technical Considerations

Anti-vimentin antibodies are among the most versatile of all commercially available antibodies. The vimentin intermediate filaments are able to survive routine tissue processing and require no specific techniques to expose the antigens. However, pretreatment with proteinase K augments the sensitivity of anti-vimentin antibodies. HIER also augments staining intensity *(16)*. Strong cytoplasmic staining can be identified within mesenchymal cells in the normal skin. This quality can be used as an appropriate positive internal control. In normal conditions, keratinocytes do not express vimentin, allowing for a good internal negative control.

Summary

Anti-vimentin antibodies have very little role in diagnostic dermato-pathology. Due to lack of specificity, positive staining does not significantly improve the accuracy of any diagnoses. There are more specific mesenchymal markers that provide much more useful information (*see* below). In our diagnostic laboratory, we do not stock this antibody. However, it does serve as a very good marker to assess for antigen preservation in tissue sections. In many laboratories, anti-vimentin antibodies serve as a positive internal control (*see* Chapter 2).

Actin (Muscle Specific/Smooth Muscle)

Introduction

Actin is an intermediate filament that is expressed by myocytes. It is a cytoskeletal protein that works in conjunction with myosin to stimulate cellular contraction *(17)*. Actin also plays a role in cellular motility and may facilitate tumor invasion *(18)*. It is also expressed by myoepithelial cells *(19)*. Focal actin expression has been demonstrated in apocrine decapitation formations and in the microvilli system in sweat glands *(17)*. In normal skin, arrector pili muscles and the smooth muscle surrounding dermal blood vessels normally express smooth muscle actin (Fig. 2). Multiple antibodies to actin have been developed and are commercially available. The most commonly used varieties are anti-smooth muscle actin and muscle-specific actin.

Diagnostic Utility

Anti-actin antibodies are especially useful in the work-up of spindle cell dermal neoplasms. As they are relatively sensitive and specific markers for muscular differentiation, a positive stain points the diagnosis in this direction (Table 1). A negative result helps to exclude muscular tumors. Actin is detected in virtually all cutaneous leiomyomas (Fig. 3) *(20)*. Actin expression is thought to be more sensitive, though possibly less specific than desmin in identifying

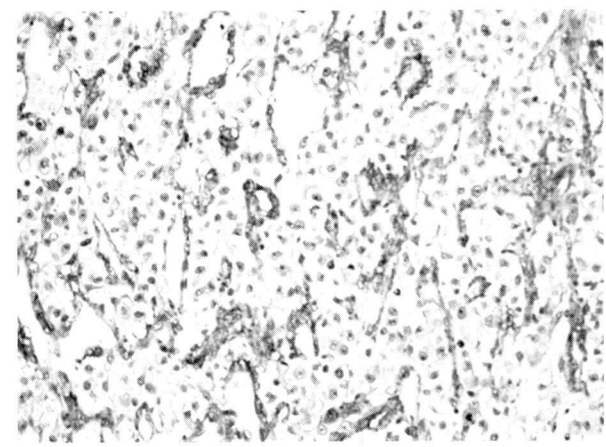

Fig. 2. Smooth muscle actin is present in cells surrounding blood vessel walls within the dermis in this vascular neoplasm.

Table 1
Essentials of Anti-Actin Antibodies*

Smooth muscle tumors	Sensitivity
Leiomyoma	100%
Glomus tumor	100%
Leiomyosarcoma	70–100%
Other tumors known to express actin	
Dermatomyofibroma	100%
Cellular neurothekeoma	50%
Granular cell dermatofibroma	10–50%
Plexiform fibrohistocytic tumor	
Infantile digital fibromatosis	
Desmoplastic melanoma	Rare

*Work in formalin-fixed, paraffin-embedded tissue. Require no pretreatment.

cutaneous leiomyosarcomas *(21–23)*. When both antigens are expressed, the diagnosis is close to certain. Glomus cells, which are modified smooth muscle cells, express actin in virtually all glomus tumors and glomangiomas *(9,24)*.

Anti-actin antibodies have been helpful in elucidating the nature of several uncommon types of cutaneous neoplasms. Anti-smooth muscle actin recognizes cells in a cellular neurothekeoma. This finding calls into question the nature of this tumor, raising the possibility

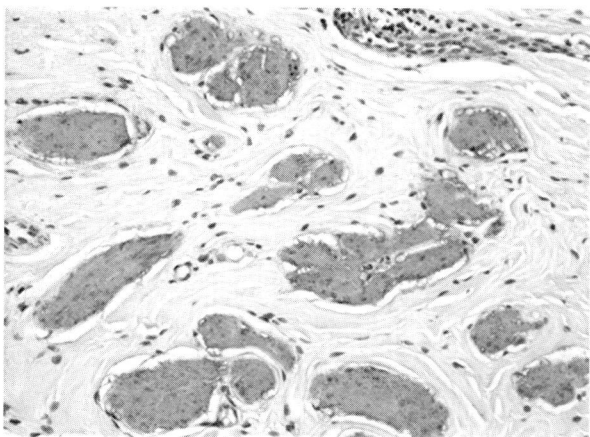

Fig. 3. Cutaneous leiomyomas strongly and diffusely express smooth muscle actin.

that it represents an epithelioid variant of a leiomyoma *(25–27)*. These neoplasms also express PGP 9.5, a neuronal marker, leaving their etiology uncertain. Dermatomyofibromas have been defined, at least in part, as myofibroblastic proliferations that express muscle specific actin and desmin (but fail to label with anti-smooth muscle actin) *(28)*. A minority of granular cell dermatofibromas also express actin *(29)*. The eosinophilic intracytoplasmic inclusions characteristic of infantile digital fibromatosis have been shown to stain intensely with anti-actin antibodies *(30)*.

Anti-actin antibodies are not completely specific for smooth muscle proliferations. Desmoplastic melanomas expressing actin have been described and may be an important differential diagnostic consideration in some cases *(31)*. However, this is an exceedingly rare finding in my experience.

Technical Considerations

There are two large categories of anti-actin antibodies. α smooth muscle actin is found only within smooth muscle cells. Monoclonal anti-α smooth muscle antibodies are useful mainly for identifying normal smooth muscle and tumors with smooth muscle differentiation. These antibodies work very well in formalin-fixed, paraffin-embedded tissue and do not require pretreatment, though sensitivity may be enhanced with trypsin or HIER pretreatment.

Anti-muscle specific actin recognizes both α and γ actins. γ Actins are present in some smooth muscle cells, but are also present in striated muscle. Anti-muscle specific actin antibodies are relatively sensitive and specific markers for all types of myogenic differentiation. The antibodies work well in formalin-fixed, paraffin-embedded tissue. HIER increases staining intensity with most anti-actin antibodies *(16)*.

Summary

Anti-actin antibodies are relatively sensitive and specific for tumors with myogenic differentiation. They are also easy to use and thus provide a useful method for confirming or refuting diagnoses of tumors with muscular differentiation. In our laboratory, there is little need to consider striated muscle proliferations on a regular basis, and we have found anti-smooth muscle actin antibodies to provide better staining results than the anti-muscle specific antibodies. For these reasons, we routinely use the anti-smooth muscle antibody in our panel of reagents, but do not stock anti-muscle specific actin.

Desmin

Introduction

Desmin is a 53 kD intermediate filament that is present in striated and smooth muscle cells. Desmin is produced by a more restricted group of cell types than is actin *(7)*. It has been localized to the filamentous bridges between Z-lines of myofibrils and sarcolemma and at the intermyofibrillar scaffolds, in conjunction with plectin *(32)*.

Diagnostic Utility

Virtually all leiomyomas express desmin (*see* Table 2) *(20)*. Anti-desmin antibodies are more variable in their staining of leiomyosarcomas (Fig. 4) *(21)*. In one study, only 80% of cutaneous leiomyosarcomas expressed desmin *(22)*. Others have suggested that desmin expression is less common in high-grade leiomyosarcomas *(33)*. The neoplastic cells in infantile digital fibromatoses, which are thought to be myofibroblasts, have been shown to express desmin, as does the same population of cells in some ossifying fibromyxoid tumors of soft parts *(30,34)*. However, other tumors of myofibroblasts such as solitary myofibromas and dermatomyofibromas have not stained with anti-desmin antibodies *(35–37)*. Primary cutaneous rhabdomyosarcomas, while extremely rare, can be identified by their desmin expression *(38,39)*. Glomus tumors, which are comprised of "modified" smooth

Table 2
Essentials of Anti-Desmin Antibodies

Smooth muscle tumors	Sensitivity
Leiomyosarcoma	80%
Leiomyoma	50–80%
Glomus tumor	0–3%

Other tumors expressing desmin
Infantile digital fibromatosis
Rhabdomyosarcoma

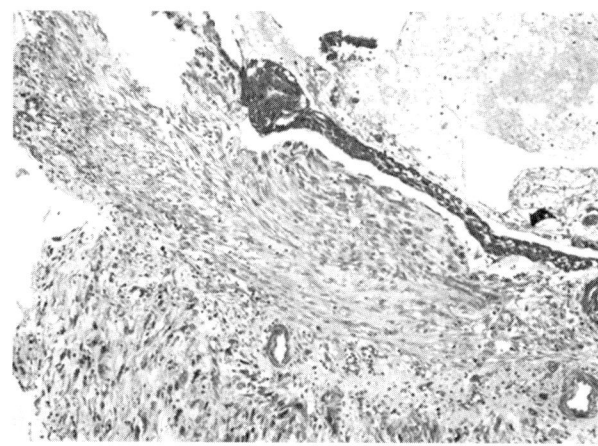

Fig. 4. Desmin expression within leiomyosarcomas may be variable and patchy.

muscle cells and express actin, do not ordinarily express desmin *(40)*. Cellular neurothekeomas, believed by some to be epithelioid leiomyomas, uniformly fail to express desmin (but stain with anti-smooth muscle actin) *(26)*.

Technical Considerations

Anti-desmin antibodies work extremely well on formalin-fixed, paraffin-embedded tissue. In general, special antigen retrieval techniques are not necessary to achieve clean and strong staining results. However, HIER has been shown to increase staining intensity *(16)*. When we use this antibody, we usually pretreat with proteinase K prior to the immunolabeling procedure.

Summary

Anti-desmin antibodies are more specific for muscle than are the anti-actin antibodies described above, but are far less sensitive. These antibodies are good antibodies that work quite well in fixed tissue, but have only a limited utility in diagnostic dermatopathology. For this reason, in our laboratory, we do not feel the need to routinely use anti-desmin antibodies. In most cases, we are able to recognize myogenic differentiation using a combination of positive staining with the anti-smooth muscle actin antibodies in conjunction with other antibodies that fail to recognize these cells.

CD34

Introduction

CD34, also known as the human progenitor cell antigen (HPCA-1), is a glycolated, 110 kD transmembrane glycoprotein. It is expressed on hematopoietic precursor cells in both the lymphoid and myeloid lines, as well as on the abluminal surfaces of vascular endothelium *(41)*. It is expressed by osteoclast precursors and by a population of cells known as dermal dendrocytes *(42)*. These cells have the ability to express either CD34 or factor XIIIa. They are involved in the cutaneous immune response and may work in conjunction with mast cells *(43)*. Clusters of spindle-shaped CD34 positive cells are found within the dermal papillae, in the follicular bulge, and around eccrine structures (Fig. 5). The exact function of these cells remains to be elucidated. They may represent a population of uncommitted mesenchymal cells *(44)*.

Diagnostic Utility

Antibodies directed against CD34 are useful in the work-up of putative vascular neoplasms (Fig. 6, Table 3). The antibody has been shown to be more sensitive than is CD31 in identifying the proliferating cells in Kaposi's sarcoma *(45)*. Some authors have reported decreased sensitivity with this antibody in detecting neoplastic endothelial cells in angiosarcomas, spindle cell hemangioendotheliomas and some cases of bacillary angiomatosis *(46)*. This is especially true within poorly differentiated, epithelioid areas of these vascular proliferations *(47)*. However, other authors have found almost uniform staining of angiosarcomas *(48)*.

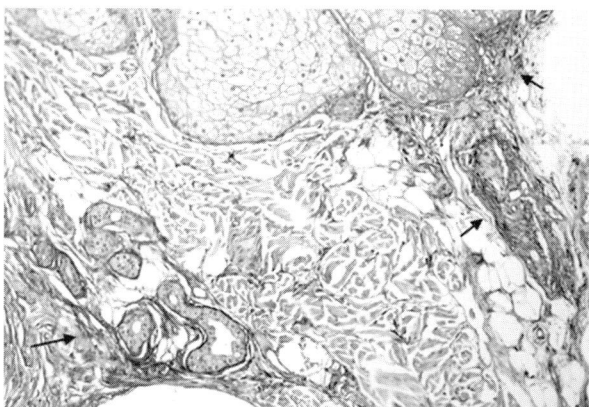

Fig. 5. Anti-CD34 identifies spindle shaped cells within the dermis, especially around eccrine ducts and hair follicles.

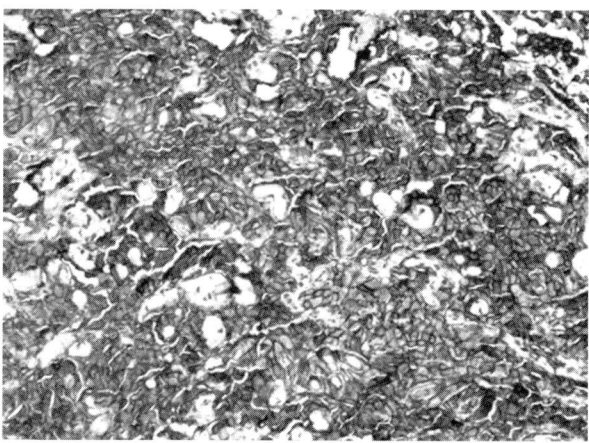

Fig. 6. CD34 is strongly expressed by endothelial cells in vascular neoplasms.

Anti- CD34 is a useful marker for identifying dermatofibrosarcoma protuberans. It strongly labels the cells in the vast majority of these tumors (Fig. 7). CD34 is not expressed ordinarily by many of the tumors in the histologic differential diagnosis such as dermatofibroma, atypical fibroxanthoma, or spindle cell melanoma *(49,50)*. Cells in giant cell fibroblastomas express CD34, reinforcing the concept that these tumors are closely related histogenetically to dermatofibrosarcoma protuberans *(51)*. Scar fibroblasts fail to express CD34, enabling staining differences to be useful in distin-

Table 3
Essentials of Anti-CD34 Antibodies*

Tumors known to express CD34	Sensitivity
Kaposi's sarcoma	100%
Lymphangioendothelioma	100%
Solitary fibrous tumor	100%
Myxoid neurothekeoma	100% (Scattered cells)
Dermatofibrosarcoma protuberans	85–100%
Angiosarcoma	21–93%
Epithelioid sarcoma	50% (weak)
Malignant peripheral nerve sheath tumor	14–20%
Leiomyosarcoma	14%
Trichilemmoma	
Acute leukemias	
Chronic leukemias	
Perineuroma	Focal
Schwannoma (Antoni B areas)	

*Work well in formalin-fixed, paraffin-embedded tissue. Require no pretreatment. Staining profile: normal dermal dendrocytes, clusters of spindle-shaped cells around hair follicles and eccrine structures.

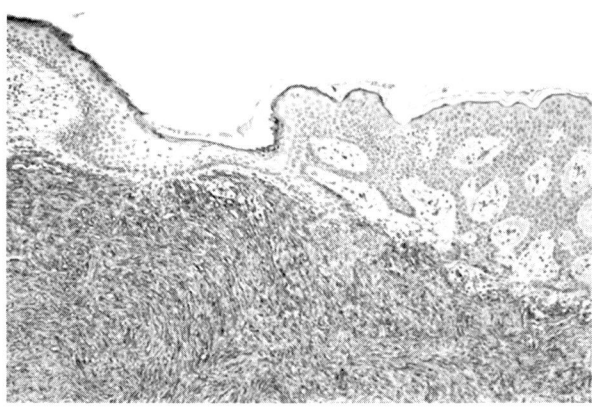

Fig. 7. CD34 expression is strong and diffuse in most dermatofibrosarcoma protuberans.

guishing residual/ recurrent dermatofibrosarcoma protuberans from scar tissue *(52)*. However, CD34 expression is not specific for dermatofibrosarcoma protuberans among spindle cell neoplasms. In addition to expression by vascular tumors discussed above, it is found on various cellular components of nerve sheath tumors, as well as by cells in solitary fibrous tumors and rare leiomyomas *(48,53–56)*.

CD34 expression by immature hematopoietic precursors can be used to advantage in the work-up of leukemia cutis. Cells in acute types of leukemia cutis stain with antibodies directed against this protein, whereas mature hematopoietic cells do not label with these antibodies *(42)*. However, as both myeloblasts and lymphoblasts express the antigen, CD34 expression is not useful in distinguishing between subtypes of acute leukemia.

CD34 is also expressed by keratinocytes that make up the follicular outer root sheath. Accordingly, tumors with differentiation towards the outer root sheath, such as trichilemmomas label with CD34. Keratinocytes in other follicular neoplasms do not express this antigen *(57)*.

Recently, desmoplastic melanomas that express CD34 have been described *(58)*.

Technical Considerations

The monoclonal CD34 antibodies work very well on paraffin-embedded, formalin-fixed tissue sections. The signal to noise ratio is enhanced with the use of trypsin digestion. HIER may also be useful, but is associated with higher background staining than is the enyzmatic pretreatment.

Summary

Anti-CD34 is a valuable reagent for an immunopathology laboratory. In conjunction with anti-CD31, it provides maximum sensitivity and specificity for identifying vascular neoplasms. It is also a very sensitive marker for recognizing dermatofibrosarcoma protuberans. Its drawback is relative lack of specificity, as it stains a wide range of spindle-cell neoplasms (Table 3). However, when used together with other, more specific markers, it offers additional support in establishing many diagnoses. The antibodies perform well on almost all fixed tissue specimens and are easy to use.

CD31

Introduction

The CD31 antigen, also known as PECAM-1 (platelet endothelial cell adhesion molecule) corresponds to the platelet glycoprotein gpIIa and is found on endothelial cells *(59)*. CD31 appears to play a vital role in the development of endothelial cell tube formation and the creation of dermal blood vessels during angiogenesis. It is a member of the immunoglobulin superfamily and interacts with filamentous actin *(60)*. The antigen is a 130-140 kD protein that functions, at least in part, as an adhesion molecule, attracting leukocytes to the endothelium *(61,62)*. CD31 is expressed on endothelial luminal membranes of blood microvasculature, as well as on both the luminal and abluminal surfaces of lymphatic endothelial cells *(41)*. CD31 is also expressed on the surfaces of platelets, monocytes, neutrophils and some B lymphocytes. Antibodies directed against CD31 were initially described in 1990, and have proven to be fairly specific markers of endothelial cell proliferations, though they also label some hematopoietic cells *(54,63)*.

Diagnostic Utility

Anti-CD31 staining was observed in 66% of vascular lesions in one large study *(54)* (Table 4). It was more sensitive than anti-CD34 in detecting angiosarcomas (Fig. 8) *(54)*. In the same study, anti-CD34 detected only 68% of vascular neoplasms. However, of significance, in the same series, anti-CD31 was not detected any nonvascular neoplasms, while anti-CD34 labeled 40% of these tumors *(54)*. Other studies have confirmed the superior sensitivity of anti-CD31 antibodies over anti-CD34 and anti-factor VIII-related antigen in labeling cells in cutaneous angiosarcomas *(64)*.

Anti-CD31 is consistently more sensitive in detecting lymphatic endothelial cells than anti-CD34 *(65,66)*. It is also a good marker for these cells in proliferative processes, labeling the vast majority of such tumors *(67)*.

In one study, CD 31 was less sensitive in marking cells in Kaposi's sarcoma than was CD34 *(54)*. Other reports have detected CD31 more frequently in cases of Kaposi's sarcoma, including the endothelial cells, stromal spindle-shaped cells, and surrounding dermal dendrocytes *(68,69)*. The weight of evidence suggests, however, that CD31 may be less sensitive overall than anti-CD34 in detecting these tumors *(64)*.

CD31 is also expressed by plasma cells. This quality may be diagnostically useful in rare situations, though there are clearly more reliable markers for identifying plasma cells (*see* Chapter 5) *(70)*.

Table 4
Essentials of Anti-CD31 Antibodies*

Vascular lining cells and neoplasms	Sensitivity
Lymphatic channels	100%
Lymphangioendothelioma	88%
Angiosarcoma	66–95%
Kaposi's sarcoma	10–75%

*Work well in formalin-fixed, paraffin-embedded tissue. Require no pretreatment.

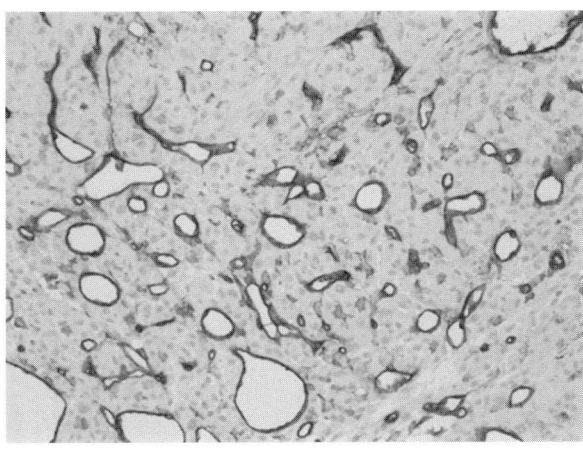

Fig. 8. Endothelial cells in most angiosarcomas express CD31 strongly and diffusely.

Technical Considerations

Antibodies directed against CD31 work extremely well on paraffin-embedded, formalin-fixed tissue sections. Pretreatment is not ordinarily necessary. However, HIER has been shown to increase the signal strength, as does pretreatment with proteinase K *(16)*.

Summary

Anti-CD31 antibodies are a first line tool for diagnosing vascular neoplasms. They enable maximum specificity for identifying endothelial cells and are also the most sensitive marker for some types of vascular neoplasms. When used in conjunction with anti-CD34 antibodies, maximum sensitivity and specificity can be achieved in narrowing down the differential diagnosis that includes vascular neoplasms.

Factor VIII-Related Antigen (von Willebrand Factor)

Introduction

Von Willebrand factor (vWF) is a 270 kD glycoprotein. It binds to platelet glycoproteins Ib, Ib/IIIa, collagen and heparin. The protein is present in platelets, megakaryocytes and endothelial cells. Commercially prepared antibodies directed against this protein have been available for a long time and were one of the first reagents available for identifying endothelial cells.

Diagnostic Utility

Anti-factor VIII-related antigen has little diagnostic utility at this time. It has been shown to be less sensitive as a marker of endothelial cell tumors than are anti-CD31 and anti-CD34 antibodies *(66)*.

Technical Considerations

Antibodies to factor VIII-related antigen (von Willebrand factor) are often plagued by high background staining, making interpretation very difficult *(66)*.

Summary

CD31 and CD34 largely have supplanted anti-factor VIII-related antigen antibodies. These antibodies are more sensitive and specific and have much cleaner staining properties. For this reason, we no longer stock these antibodies in our laboratory.

Factor XIIIa

Introduction

Factor XIIIa is a component of the coagulation cascade. It is expressed by a subpopulation of spindle shaped cells in the dermis and is present in the rough endoplasmic reticulum of these cells (Fig. 9) *(71)*. This population of cells is involved in antigen presentation and is derived from the bone marrow *(72)*. These cells also express HLA-DR, LFA-1 and multiple macrophage markers. They do not express CD1a, unlike Langherhans cells *(72)*. The exact relationship between factor XIIIa positive cells and similar appearing CD34 positive, factor XIIIa negative cells in the dermis is not yet fully understood.

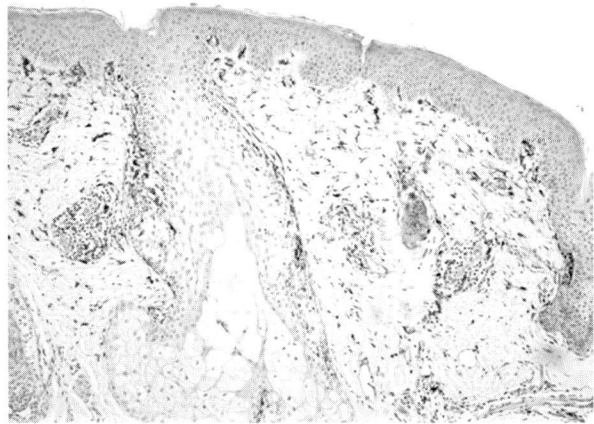

Fig. 9. Factor XIIIa positive cells are present diffusely throughout the dermis of normal skin.

Diagnostic Utility

Anti-factor XIIIa antibodies have a very limited number of conditions for which they are diagnostically useful. The tumor cells in dermatofibromas strongly express factor XIIIa in almost all cases (Fig. 10) *(49,73)*. This is in contrast to dermatofibrosarcoma protuberans, whose cells are almost always negative with this marker. The cells in various other dermal conditions such as fibrous papules and pleomorphic fibromas have been shown to express factor XIIIa (Fig. 11), but while these observations provide interesting insights into pathogenesis and disease processes, they do not provide any additional diagnostic help *(74)*. Spindle shaped cells in other fibrotic dermal processes including cells in scars and keloids do not express factor XIIIa *(75)*.

Technical Considerations

Anti-factor XIIIa works on formalin-fixed, paraffin-embedded tissue. Enyzmatic digestion or HIER for antigen retrieval is necessary in order to maximize sensitivity. In our laboratory, we pretreat with proteinase K prior to the immunolabeling procedure.

Summary

Anti-factor XIIIa antibodies play a limited role in diagnostic dermatopathology. The antibody is particularly useful in the distinction

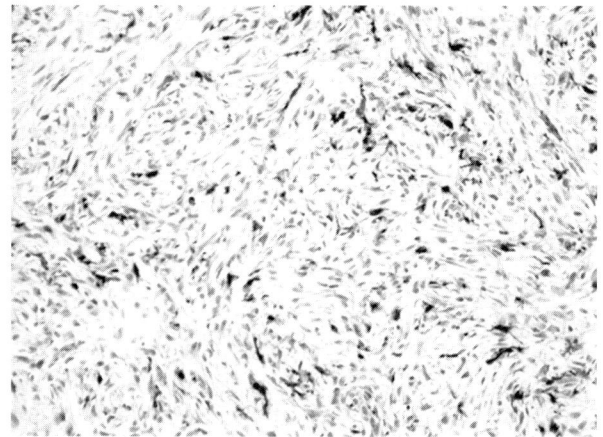

Fig. 10. Many cells express factor XIIIa in dermatofibromas.

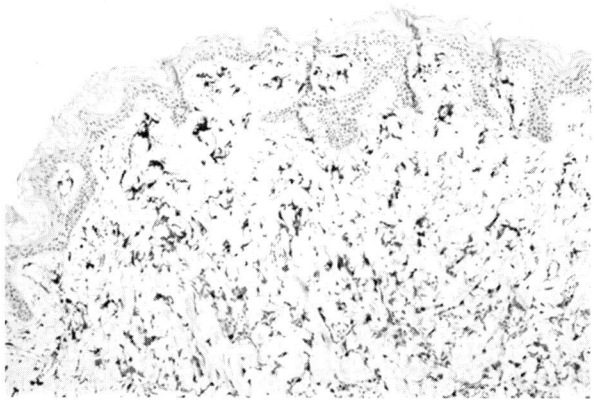

Fig. 11. The large, atypical and stellate cells in pleomorphic fibromas express factor XIIIa.

between dermatofibroma and dermatofibrosarcoma protuberans when routine histology is not diagnostic. However, as this differential diagnosis is not usually difficult to resolve using routine sections, and as there are limited alternative uses for this reagent, it is not essential for a dermatopathology laboratory to stock this antibody. We use it as part of the panel of antibodies in the work-ups of dermatofibrosarcoma protuberans and atypical fibroxanthoma.

References

1. Rappersberger, K., Binder, M., Zonzits, E., Hornick, U., and Wolff, K. (1990) Immunogold staining of intermediate-sized filaments of the vimentin type in human skin: a postembedding immunoelectron microscopic study. *J. Invest. Dermatol.* **94,** 700–705.

2. Gabbiani, G., Kaanci, Y., Barazzone, P., and Franke, W. W. (1981) Immunochemical identification of intermediate-sized filaments in human neoplastic cells. A diagnostic aid for the surgical pathologist. *Am. J. Pathol.* **104,** 206–216.

3. Osborn, M. (1983) Intermediate filaments as histologic markers: an overview. *J. Invest. Dermatol.* **81 (1 Suppl),** 104s–109s.

4. Huszar, M., KHalkin, H., Herczeg, E., Bubis, J., and Gieger, B. (1983) Use of antibodies to intermediate filaments in the diagnosis of metastatic amelanotic malignant melanoma. *Hum. Pathol.* **14,** 1006–1008.

5. Caselitz, J., Janner, M., Breitbart, E., Weber, K., and Osborn, M. (1983) Malignant melanomas contain only the vimentin type of intermediate filaments. *Virchows Arch. A Pathol. Anat. Histopathol.* **400,** 43–51.

6. Mahrle, G., Bolling, R., Osborn, M., and Weber, K. (1983) Intermediate filaments of the vimentin and prekeratin type in human epidermis. *J. Invest. Dermatol.* **81,** 46–48.

7. Miettinen, M., Lehto, V. P., and Virtanen, I. (1985) Antibodies to intermediate filament proteins. The differential diagnosis of cutaneous tumors. *Arch. Dermatol.* **121,** 736–741.

8. Eckert, F., Burg, G., Braun-Falco, O., Schmid, U., and Gloor, F. (1988) Immunostaining in aypical fibroxanthoma of the skin. *Pathol. Res. Pract.* **184,** 27–34.

9. Dervan, P. A., Tobbia, I. N., Casey, M., O'Loughlin, J., and O'Brien, M. (1989) Glomus tumors: an immunohistochemical profile of 11 cases. *Histopathology* **14,** 483–491.

10. Smith, K. J., Skelton, H. G., III, Morgan, A. M., Barrett, T. L., and Lupton, G. P. (1992) Spindle cell neoplasms coexpressing cytokeratin and vimentin (metaplastic squamous cell carcinomas). *J. Cutan. Pathol.* **19,** 286–293.

11. Gray, Y., Robidoux, H. J., Farrell, D. S., and Robinson-Bostom, L. (2001) Squamous cell carcinoma detected by high-molecular-weight cytokeratin immunostaining mimicking atypical fibroxanthoma. *Arch. Pathol. Lab. Med.* **125,** 799–802.

12. Iyer, P. V. and Leong, A. S. (1992) Poorly differentiated squamous cell carcinomas of the skin can express vimentin. *J. Cutan. Pathol.* **19,** 34–39.

13. Swanson, S. A., Cooper, P. H., Mills, S. E., and Wick, M. R. (1988) Lymphoepithelioma-like carcinoma of the skin. *Mod. Pathol.* **1,** 359–365.

14. Santa Cruz, D. J., Barr, R. J., and Headington, J. T. (1991) Cutaneous lymphadenoma. *Am. J. Surg. Pathol.* **15,** 101–110.

15. Sangueza, O. P., Meshul, C. K., Sangueza, P., and Mendoza, R. (1992) Rhabdoid tumor of the skin. *Int. J. Dermatol.* **31,** 484–487.

16. Gown, A. M., de Wever, N., and Battifora, H. 1993, Microwave-based antigenic unmasking. A revolutionary new technique for routine immunohistochemistry. *Appl. Immunohistochem.* **1,** 256–266.

17. Metzler, G., Shaumburg-Lever, G., Fehrenbacher, B., and Moller, H. (1992) Ultrastructural localization of actin in normal human skin. *Arch. Dermatol. Res.* **284,** 242–245.

18. Christian, M. M., Moy, R. L., Wagner, R. F., and Yen-Moore, A. (2001) A correlation of alpha-smooth muscle actin and invasion in micronodular basal cell carcinoma. *Dermatol. Surg.* **27,** 441–445.

19. Eckert, F., Betke, M., Schmoeckel, C., Neuweiler, J., and Schmid, U. (1992) Myoepithelial differentiation in benign sweat gland tumors. Demonstrated by a monoclonal antibody to alpha-smooth muscle actin. *J. Cutan. Pathol.* **19,** 294–301.

20. Yokoyama, R., Hashimoto, H., Daimaru, Y., and Enjoji, M. (1987) Superficial leiomyomas. A clinicopathologic study of 34 cases. *Act. Pathol. Jpn.* **37,** 1415–1422.

21. Lundgren, L., Kindblom, L. G., Seidal, T., and Angervall, L. (1991) Intermediate and fine cytofilaments in cutaneous and subcutaneous leiomyosarcomas. *APMIS* **99,** 820–828.

22. Kaddu, S., Beham, A., Cerroni, L., Humer-Fuchs, U., Salmhofer, W., Kerl, H., and Soyer, H. P. (1997) Cutaneous leiomyosarcoma. *Am. J. Surg. Pathol.* **21,** 979–987.

23. Hashimoto, H., Daimaru, Y., Tsuneyoshi, M., and Enjoji, M. (1986) Leiomyosarcoma of the external soft tissues. A clinicopatohlogic, immunohistochemical, and electron microscopic study. *Cancer* **57,** 2077–2088.

24. Kaye, V. M. and Dehner, L. P. (1991) Cutaneous glomus tumor. A comparative immunohistochemical study with pseudoangiomatous intradermal melanocytic nevi. *Am. J. Dermatopathol.* **13,** 2–6.

25. Chatelain, D., Ricard, J., Colombat, M., Ghighi, C., Thelu, F., Cordonnier, C., Gontier, M. F., and Sevestre, H. (2000) Cellular neurothekeoma, a rare cutaneous tumor. Anatomoclinical and immunohistochemical study of 2 cases. *Ann. Pathol.* **20,** 225–227.

26. Calonje, E., Wilson-Jones, E., Smith, N. P., and Fletcher, C. D. (1992) Cellular 'neurothekeoma': an epithelioid variant of pilar leiomyoma? Morphological and immunohistochemical analysis of a series. *Histopathology* **20,** 397–404.

27. Argenyi, Z. B., LeBoit, P. E., Santa Cruz, D., Swanson, P. E., and Kutzner, H. (1993) Nerve sheath myxoma (neurothekeoma) of the skin: light microscopic and immunohistochemical reappraisal of the cellular variant. *J. Cutan. Pathol.* **20,** 294–303.

28. Kamino, H., Reddy, V. B., Gero, M., and Greco, M. A. (1992) Dermatomyofibroma. A benign cutaneous, plaque-like proliferation of fibroblasts and myofibrolasts in young adults. *J. Cutan. Pathol.* **19,** 85–93.

29. Zelger, B. G., Steiner, H., Kutzner, H., Rutten, A., and Zelger, B. (1997) Granular cell dermatofibroma. *Histopathology* **31,** 258–262.

30. Choi, K. C., Hashimoto, H., Setoyama, M., Kagetsu, N., Tronnier, M., and Sturman, S. (1990) Infantile digital fibromatosis. Immunohistochemical and immunoelectron microscopic studies. *J. Cutan. Pathol.* **17,** 225–232.

31. Riccioni, L., Di Tommaso, L., and Collina, G. (1999) Actin-rich desmoplastic malignant melanoma: report of three cases. *Am. J. Dermatopathol.* **21,** 537–541.

32. Schroder, R., Warlo, I., Herrmann, H., van der Ven, P. F., Klasen, C., Blumcke, I., Mundegar, R. R., Furst, D. O., Goebel, H. H., and Magin, T. M. (1999) Immunogold EM reveals a close association of plectin and the desmin cytoskeleton in human skeletal muscle. *Eur. J. Cell. Biol.* **78,** 288–295.

33. Oliver, G. F., Reiman, H. M., Gonchoroff, N. J., Muller, S. A., and Umbert, I. J. (1991) Cutaneous and subcutaneous leiomyosarcoma: a clinicopathological review of 14 cases with reference to antidesmin staining and nuclear DNA patterns studied by flow cytometry. *Brit. J. Dermatol.* **124,** 252–257.

34. Fukunaga, M., Ushigome, S., and Ishikawa, E. (1994) Ossifying subcutaneous tumor with myofibroblastic differentiation: a variant of ossifying fibromyxoid tumor of soft parts? *Path. Int.* **44,** 727–734.

35. Beham, A., Badve, S., Suster, S., and Fletcher, C. D. (1993) Solitary myofibroma in adults: clinicopathological analysis of a series. *Histopathology* **22,** 335–341.

36. Colome, M. I. and Sanchez, R. L. (1994) Dermatomyofibroma: report of two cases. *J. Cutan. Pathol.* **21,** 371–376.

37. Zelger, B. W., Zelger, B. G., and Rappersberger, K. (1997) Prominent myofibroblastic differentiation. A pitfall in the diagnosis of dermatofibroma. *Am. J. Dermatopathol.* **19,** 138–146.

38. Chang, Y., Dehner, L. P., and Egbert, B. M. (1990) Primary cutaneous rhabdomyosarcoma. *Am. J. Surg. Pathol.* **14,** 977–982.

39. Schmidt, D., Fletcher, C. D., and Harms, D. (1993) Rhabdomyosarcomas with primary presentation in the skin. *Pathol. Res. Pract.* **189,** 422–427.

40. Miettinen, M., Lehto, V. P., and Virtanen, I. (1983) Glomus tumor cels: evaluation of smooth muscle and endothelial cell properties. *Virchows Arch. B Cell. Pathol. Incl. Mol. Pathol.* **43,** 139–149.

41. Sauter, B., Foedinger, D., Sterniczky, B., Wolff, K., and Rappersberger, K. (1998) Immunoelectron microscopic characterization of human dermal lymphatic microvascular endothelial cells. Differential expression of CD31, CD34, and type IV collagen with lymphatic endothelial cells vs. blood capillary endothelial cells in normal human skin, lymphangioma, and hemangioma in situ. *J. Histochem. Cytochem.* **46,** 165–176.

42. Silvestri, F., Banavali, S., Baccarani, M., and Preisler, H. D. (1992) The CD34 hemopoietic progenitor cell associated antigen: biology and clinical applications. *Haematologica* **77,** 265–273.

43. Sueki, H., Whitaker, D. C., Buchsbaum, M., and Murphy, G. F. (1993) Novel interaction between dermal dendrocytes and mast cells in human skin. Implications for hemostasis and matrix repair. *Lab. Invest.* **69,** 160–172.

44. Narvaez, D., Kanitakis, J., Faure, M., and Claudy, A. (1996) Immunhistochemical study of CD34-positive dendritic cells of human dermis. *Am. J. Dermatopathol.* **18,** 283–288.

45. Nickoloff, B. J. (1991) The human progenitor cell antigen (CD34) is localized on endothelial cells, dermal dendritic cells, and perifollicular cells in formalin-fixed normal skin, and on proliferating endothelial cells and stromal spindle-shaped cells in Kaposi's sarcoma. *Arch. Dermatol.* **127,** 523–529.

46. Suster, S. and Wong, T. Y. (1994) On the discriminatory value of anti-HPCA-1 (CD34) in the differential diagnosis of benign and malignant cutaneous vascular proliferations. *Am. J. Dermatopathol.* **16,** 355–363.

47. Poblet, E., Gonzalez-Palacios, F., and Jimenez, F. J. (1996) Different immunoreactivity of endothelial markers in well and poorly differentiated areas of angiosarcomas. *Virchows Arch.* **428,** 217–221.

48. Traweek, S. T., Kandlaft, P. L., Mehta, P., and Battifora, H. (1991) The human hamtopoietic progenitor cell antigen (CD34) in vascular neoplasia. *Am. J. Clin. Pathol.* **96,** 25–31.

49. Altman, D. A., Nickoloff, B. J., and Fivenson, D. P. (1993) Differential expression of factor XIIIa and CD34 in cutaneous mesenchymal tumors. *J. Cutan. Pathol.* **20,** 154–158.

50. Kutzner, H. (1993) Expression of the human progenitor cell antigen (HPCA-1) distinguishes dermatofibrosarcoma protuberans from fibrous histiocytoma in formalin-fixed, paraffin-embedded tissue. *J. Am. Acad. Dermatol.* **28,** 613–617.

51. Weiss, S. W. and Nickoloff, B. J. (1993) CD-34 is expressed by a distinctive cell population in peripheral nerve, nerve sheath tumors, and related lesions. *Am. J. Surg. Pathol.* **17,** 1039–1045.

52. Prieto, V., Reed, J. A., and Shea, C. R. (1994) CD34 immunoreactivity distinguishes between scar tissue and residual tumor in re-excisional specimens of dermatofibrosarcoma protuberans. *J. Cutan. Pathol.* **21,** 324–329.

53. Okamura, J. M., Barr, R. J., and Battifora, H. (1997) Solitary fibrous tumor of the skin. *Am. J. Dermatopathol.* **19,** 515–518.

54. DeYoung, B. R., Swanson, P. E., Argenyi, Z. B., Ritter, J. H., Fitzgibbon, J. F., Stahl, D. J., et al. (1995) CD31 immunoreactivity in mesenchymal neoplasms of the skin and subcutis: report of 145 cases and review of putative immunohistochemical markers of endothelial differentiation. *J. Cutan. Pathol.* **22,** 215–222.

55. Laskin, W. B., Fetsch, J. F., and Miettinen, M. (2000) The "neurothekeoma": immunohistochemical analysis distinguishes the true nerve sheath myxoma from its mimics. *Hum. Pathol.* **31,** 1230–1241.

56. Hirose, T., Scheithauer, B. W., and Sano, T. (1998) Perineural malignant peripheral nerve sheath tumor (MPNST): a clinicopathologic, immuonhistochemical, and ultrastructural study of seven cases. *Am. J. Surg. Pathol.* **22,** 1368–1378.

57. Poblet, E., Jimenez-Acosta, F., and Rocamora, A. (1994) QBEND/10 (anti-CD34 antibody) in external root sheath cells and follicular tumors. *J. Cutan. Pathol.* **21,** 224–228.

58. Hoang, M. P., Selim, M. A., Burchette, J. L., and Shea, C. R. (2001) CD34 expression in desmplastic melanoma. *J. Cutan. Pathol.* **28,** 508–512.

59. Bordessoule, D., Jones, M., Gatter, K. C., and Mason, D. Y. (1993) Immunohistological patterns of myeloid antigens: tissue distribution of CD13, CD14, CD16, CD31, CD36, CD65, CD66 and CD67. *Brit. J. Haematol.* **83,** 370–383.

60. Matsumura, T., Wolff, K., and Petzelbauer, P. (1997) Endothelial cell tube formation depends on cadherin 5 and CD31 interactions with filamentous actin. *J. Immunol.* **158,** 3408–3416.

61. Newman, P. J., Berndt, M. C., Gorski, J., White, G. C., 2nd, Lyman, S., Paddoci, C., and Muller, W. A. (1990) PECAM-1 (CD31) cloning and relation to adhesion molecules of the immunoglobulin gene superfamily. *Science* **247,** 1219–1222.

62. DeLisser, H. M., BNewman, P. J., and Albelda, S. M. (1993) Platelet endothelial cell adhesion molecule. *Curr. Top. Microbiol. Immunol.* **184,** 37–45.

63. Parums, D. V., Cordell, J. L., Micklem, K., Heryet, A. R., Gatter, K. C., and Mason, D. Y. (1990) JC70: a new monoclonal antibody that detects vascular endothelium associated antigen on routinely processed tissue sections. *J. Clin. Pathol.* **43,** 752–757.

64. Orchard, G. E., Zelger, B., Jones, E. W., and Jones, R. R. (1996) An immunocytochemical assessment of 19 cases of cutaneous angiosarcoma. *Histopathology* **28,** 235–240.

65. Ramani, P. and Shah, A. (1993) Lymphangiomatosis. Histologic and immunohistochemical analysis of four cases. *Am. J. Surg. Pathol.* **17,** 329–335.

66. Miettinen, M., Lindenmayer, A. E., and Chaubal, A. (1994) Endothelial cell markers CD31, CD34, and BNH9 antibody to H- and Y- antigens—evaluation of their specificity and sensitivity in the diagnosis of vascular tumors and comparison with von Willebrand factor. *Mod. Pathol.* **7,** 82–90.

67. Guillou, L. and Fletcher, C. D. (2000) Benign lymphangioendothelioma (acquired progressive lymphangioma): a lesion not to be confused with well-differentiated angiosarcoma and patch stage Kaposi's sarcoma: clinicopathologic analysis of a series. *Am. J. Surg. Pathol.* **24,** 1047–1057.

68. Nickoloff, B. J. (1993) PECAM-1 (CD31) is expressed on proliferating endothelial cells, stromal spindle-shaped cells, and dermal dendrocytes in Kaposi's sarcoma. *Arch. Dermatol.* **129,** 250–251.

69. Uccini, S., Ruco, L. P., Monardo, F., Stoppacciaro, A., Dejana, E., La Parola, I. L., Cerimele, D., and Baroni, C. D. (1994) Co-expression of endothelial cell and macrophage antigens in Kaposi's sarcoma cells. *J. Pathol.* **173,** 23–31.

70. Wang, E., Pierre, K. S., Peng, S.-K., and Shitabata, P. (2001) A cutaneous plasmacytoma masquerades as skin appendage tumors and soft tissue neoplasms (abstract). *J. Cutan. Pathol.* **28,** 552.

71. Schaumburg-Lever, G., Gehring, B., and Kaiserling, E. (1994) Ultrastructural localization of factor XIIIa. *J. Cutan. Pathol.* **21,** 129–134.

72. Cerio, R., Griffiths, C. E., Cooper, K. D., Nickoloff, B. J., and Headington, J. T. (1989) Characterization of factor XIIIa positive dermal dendritic cells in normal and inflamed skin. Brit. J. Dermatol. 121, 421–431.

73. Cerio, R., Spaull, J., and Jones, E. W. (1989) Histiocytoma cutis: a tumour of dermal dendrocytes (dermal dendrocytoma). Brit. J. Dermatol. 120, 197–206.

74. Nemeth, A. J., Penneys, N. S., and Bernstein, H. B. (1988) Fibrous papule: a tumor of fibrohistiocytic cells that contain factor XIIIa. *J. Am. Acad. Dermatol.* **19,** 1102–1106.

75. Cerio, R., Spaull, J., Oliver, G. F., and Jones, E. W. (1990) A study of factor XIIIa and MAC 387 immunolabeling in normal and pathological skin. *Am. J. Dermatopathol.* **12,** 221–233.

5 Hematopoietic Markers

CD45RB (Leukocyte Common Antigen)
Introduction

Leukocyte common antigen (LCA) is a membrane protein that is restricted largely to leukocytes *(1)*. It has two intracellular catalytic domains and is part of the tyrosine phosphatase family *(2)*. The leukocyte common antigen family of proteins is comprised of enzymes thought to play a role in cellular activation *(3)*. There are more specific isoforms of this antigen, namely CD45RA, expressed by "naïve" T cells, and CD45RO, expressed by "memory" T cells *(4)*. There are specific antibodies directed against these isoforms. The following discussion addresses the antibodies directed against the broader CD45RB antigens.

Diagnostic Utility

Anti-LCA antibody routinely labels B and T lymphocytes. It localizes to the cellular membranes and focally to the cytoplasm (Fig. 1). Monocytes and mast cells also express this protein. However, myeloid cells, megakaryocytes and erythrocytes do not. Reed-Sternberg cells only variably express LCA. It is important to note that plasma cells do not express LCA *(1)*. Only membrane staining of the cells should be considered as true staining. Occasional granular staining within the cytoplasm can be seen in other cell types and is not specific.

Technical Considerations

Anti-LCA antibodies are readily available and generally easy to use. They work extremely well on formalin-fixed, paraffin-embedded tissue and do not require any type of pretreatment to expose the antigenic sites.

Summary

There is only limited utility for anti-LCA antibodies in diagnostic dermatopathology. In the vast majority of cases, it is possible to identify cells as being hematopoietic without resorting to antibody

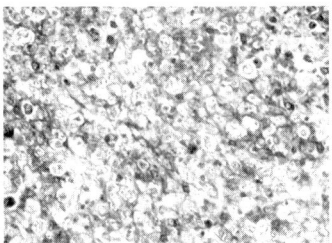

Fig. 1. Leukocyte common antigen is strongly expressed by the vast majority of hematopoietic cells.

labeling. However, in the rare cases when it is difficult to make this distinction, this antibody may be useful. It should be noted that in some types of large cell lymphomas and plasma cell proliferations, LCA might not be expressed by neoplastic leukocytes, further diminishing the utility of this marker.

B Lymphocyte Markers
Kappa and Lambda Light Chains

INTRODUCTION

In the circulating blood, approx 70% of B lymphocytes produce kappa light chains and the other 30% lambda light chains. This ratio is similar to that seen in lymphocytes present within the dermis. This biologic property can be used to assess for the presence of clonality in B cell infiltrates within the skin.

DIAGNOSTIC UTILITY

Antibodies directed against kappa and lambda light chains could be difficult to interpret. The antibodies are nonspecifically adsorbed by dermal collagen, giving a very high background "blush" staining in many cases (Fig. 2). However, the staining appears much cleaner in densely cellular areas, as there is little collagen to adsorb the antibody, and interpretation is not difficult if skin biopsies contain sufficient masses of lymphocytes (Fig. 3). In general, a case for monoclonality can be made if there is a ratio of 10:1 or greater between kappa and lambda expressing cells in a lymphoid infiltrate *(5)*. Use of anti-kappa and anti-lambda antibodies to assess monoclonality is especially useful in establishing a diagnosis of

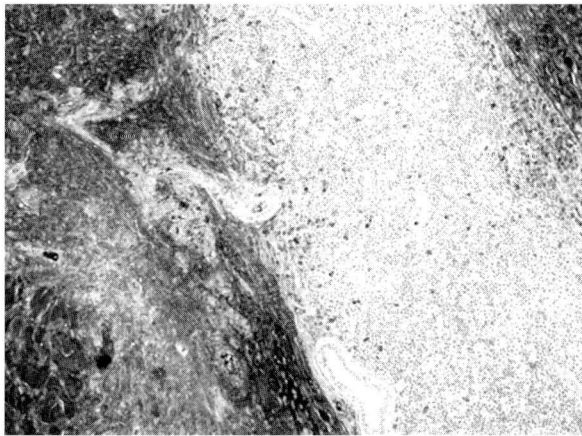

Fig. 2. Anti-kappa antibodies demonstrating cellular staining along with non-specific high background staining of surrounding dermal collagen.

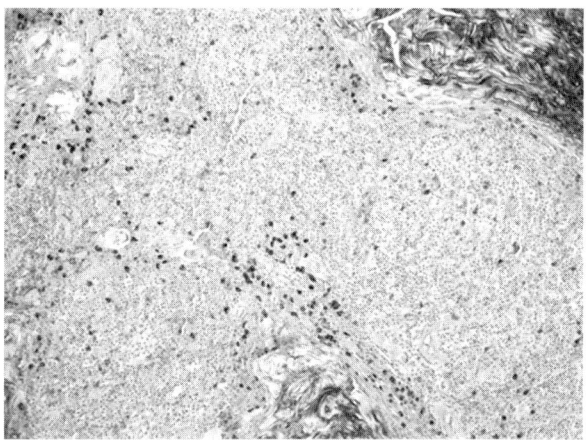

Fig. 3. In more cellular areas, strong staining of individual cells with anti-lambda antibodies is easily interpreted.

marginal zone lymphoma, which may be very difficult to do on routine tissue sections (Table 1) *(6)*.

TECHNICAL CONSIDERATIONS

As mentioned above, while antibodies to kappa and lambda light chains work well in formalin-fixed, paraffin-embedded tissue sections, there are some limitations when using these antibodies on skin sections. Collagen fibers nonspecifically adsorb the antibodies, making tissue sections appear dirty and providing a high background. In cases with only a pauci-cellular infiltrate of hematopoietic cells, this nonspecific staining precludes interpretation. However, in densely cellular dermal infiltrates, the desired staining patterns can be readily distinguished from the nonspecific staining and the antibodies can be very useful in detecting light chain restriction. HIER has been shown to increase staining intensity with these antibodies *(7)*. In our laboratory, we routinely pretreat with proteinase K prior to initiating the immunolabeling procedure.

SUMMARY

Anti-kappa and anti-light chain antibodies, when used together, are very helpful in detecting clonality of B lymphocytes or a plasmacellular population of cells within the dermis.

CD10

INTRODUCTION

CD10 also known as cALLA is a marker for immature B lymphocytes. It was initially identified as a very early marker expressed by lymphoblastic leukemia cells *(8)*. It is one of many exopeptidases that is involved in activation and deactivation of peptides.

DIAGNOSTIC UTILITY

CD10 functions as a useful marker for B-lineage lymphomas. However, it is less specific than was originally thought and can be seen on a wider range of leukemias and lymphomas *(8)*. CD10 is also expressed by some follicular center cell lymphocytes and thus can serve as an additional marker of follicular center cell lymphomas *(9)*. Cells in small cleaved, mixed small and large cell, and large cell lymphomas, as well as small noncleaved (Burkitts) lymphomas (Table 1) express CD10 *(10)*. However, it should be noted that the majority of cutaneous B cell lymphomas fail to express CD10, as they are marginal zone lymphomas, and not of follicular center cell origin. Mantle zone lymphomas are B cell neoplasms that uniformly fail to stain with anti-CD10 antibody *(11)*. Further, many of the primary cutaneous follicular center cell lymphomas also fail to express CD10 *(12)*.

Table 1
Immunologic Work-Up of a B Cell Lymphoma

Follicular center cell lymphoma
  CD20 + (often lost in large cell B cell lymphomas)
  CD43 ±
  CD3 −
  Kappa and lambda light chains–restricted expression
  CD10 + (optional)
  CD79a + (optional)
Marginal zone lymphoma (immunocytoma)
  CD20 +
  CD43 −
  CD3 −
  Kappa and lambda light chains–restricted expression
  CD10 − (optional)
  CD79a −
Mantle zone lymphoma
  CD20 +
  CD43 −
  CD5 +
  CD10 −
  CD79a +
  Bcl-2 −

Anti-CD10 antibodies are not absolutely specific for hematopoietic cells. Almost half of melanomas (primary and metastatic) label with this antibody *(13)*.

TECHNICAL CONSIDERATIONS

Anti-CD10 antibodies that survive routine tissue processing are readily available and work adequately with little practice. Technologic problems do not present a rate-limiting step for the use of this antibody in routine practice.

SUMMARY

There is little use for anti-CD10 antibodies in routine diagnostic dermatopathology. In cases where unusual types of cutaneous lymphoma and leukemia arc being considered, the addition of this antibody to the panel may be helpful. However, unless the laboratory sees a high volume of cutaneous lymphomas, it may not be practical to keep this antibody in stock.

CD20

INTRODUCTION

CD20 is a surface antigen that is expressed by the vast majority of immature and mature B lymphocytes *(14)*. It has four membrane spanning domains and may function as a regulator of transmembrane calcium conductance. In this way, it may be essential in B cell activation, proliferation and/or differentiation *(15)*.

DIAGNOSTIC UTILITY

CD20 serves as a good initial screening marker in defining subpopulations of lymphocytes *(see* Table 1). In the normal skin, there are very few B lymphocytes. In some conditions giving rise to cutaneous lymphoid hyperplasia, recapitulation of nodal architecture as evidenced by follicular centers and mantle zones may be present. Follicular centers are accentuated by strong staining of cells with anti-CD20 antibodies (Fig. 4) *(16)*.

In cutaneous B cell lymphomas of small or mixed-cell types, CD20 is almost always expressed diffusely throughout (17). Loss of CD20 is sometimes observed in large cell B cell lymphomas.

TECHNICAL CONSIDERATIONS

Anti-CD20 antibodies are commercially available. They work extremely well in formalin-fixed, paraffin-embedded tissue sections and do not ordinarily require the tissue sections to be pretreated. HIER has been shown to increase staining intensity with this antibody *(7)*.

SUMMARY

CD20 is currently the best overall marker for B lymphocytes. These cells are not often present in large numbers within the dermis, except in some cases of cutaneous lymphoid hyperplasia. Thus, the presence of sheets of lymphocytes expressing CD20 that are not forming germinal centers is strong evidence in favor of a cutaneous lymphoma.

CD79a

INTRODUCTION

CD79 has two components known as CD79a and CD79b. The antigen is expressed by B lymphocytes prior to the expression of immunoglobulins. It is present in B cells throughout maturation, but disappears as they evolve into plasma cells *(18)*.

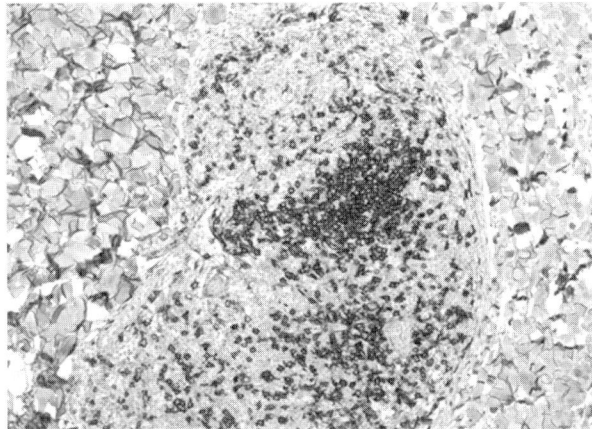

Fig. 4. B cells in reactive germinal centers express CD20. A surrounding collarette of CD20 negative T cells is also seen.

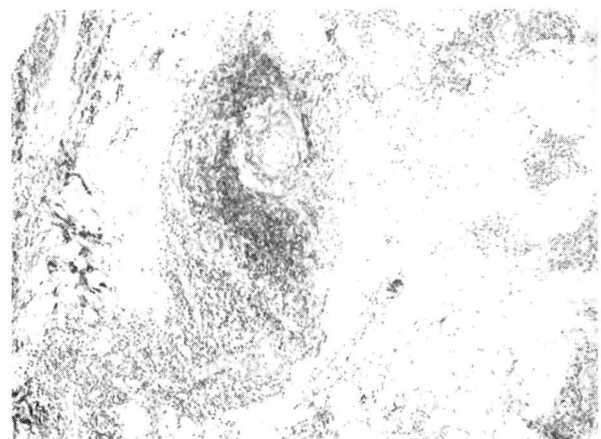

Fig. 5. CD79a is seen on B cells in this case of cutaneous lymphoid hyperplasia. The CD79a negative cells are T cells (that labeled with CD3, not shown).

DIAGNOSTIC UTILITY

Anti-CD79a antibodies are useful in distinguishing B from T cell infiltrates (Fig. 5) (Table 1). As all B lymphocytes with the exception of plasma cells express this antigen, it is relatively sensitive. The antigen has not been reported on T lymphocytes, making it very specific. It can be used as a good marker for B type of acute lymphoblastic leukemias, since the antigen is present in these immature precursor cells, as well *(18)*.

For most B cell lymphomas, anti-CD20 works as a first line marker. However, in some large cell lymphomas, the CD20 antigen may be lost. In these cases, anti-CD79a, which is usually preserved, is very helpful in establishing the B lineage of the tumor cells *(18)*.

Cells in hairy cell leukemia express CD79a *(19)*.

Technical Considerations

There are commercially available antibodies to CD79a that recognize the antigen on routinely processed tissue. Antigen retrieval techniques such as HIER markedly augment the staining intensity of these antibodies.

Summary

In most cases, anti-CD20 is sufficient to establish B cell lineage in cutaneous lymphoid infiltrates. However, in many ways, CD79a is a more useful marker, as earlier precursor cells express it than do CD20, as well as cells later in development. While it is lost in plasma cells, this is also the case with CD20. There is probably no need for the usual dermatopathology laboratory to keep both antibodies, as the indications for one over the other are relatively limited. For most laboratories, there is more extensive experience using the CD20 antibodies, but as the more recently developed anti-CD79a antibodies become more widely used, they may supplant the anti-CD20 as the gold standard for identifying B lymphocytes.

Bcl-2

Introduction

Bcl-2 is a protein that functions as a cellular anti-apoptosis signal. It is constituitively expressed by basal keratinocytes and melanocytes within the skin, but not within keratinocytes above the basal layer *(20)*. T lymphocytes also express bcl-2 protein in all conditions. However, bcl-2 protein is not ordinarily expressed by reactive B lymphocytes. Its expression has been shown to be upregulated in nodal follicular lymphomas due to a clonally rearranged gene *(20)*.

Diagnostic Utility

Anti-bcl-2 was initially thought to be a good marker for cutaneous B cell lymphomas, based upon the observation that reactive B cell did

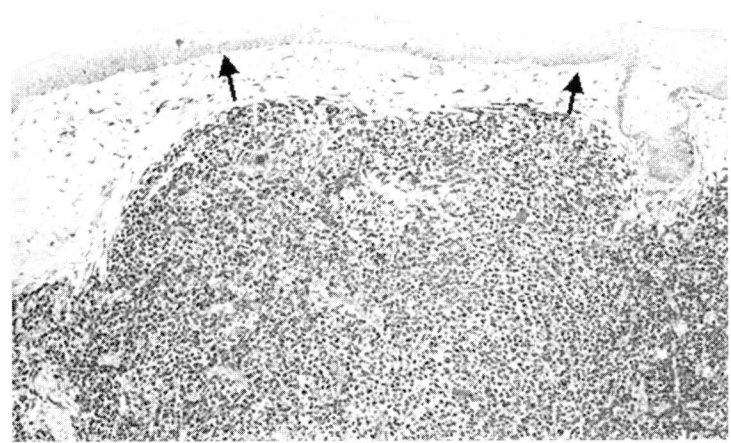

Fig. 6. Cells in this primary cutaneous follicular center cell lymphoma strongly expressed bcl-2.

not express the protein and neoplastic follicular center cells did. However, recent literature has called into question this supposition. In one study, the cells in 58% of B cell lymphomas expressed this protein, but bcl-2 was also found in 33% of cases of cutaneous lymphoid hyperplasia (Fig. 6). However, on closer examination, neoplastic follicles expressed bcl-2 in 66% of cases, while it was not found in the germinal centers in any of the cases of reactive lymphoid hyperplasia *(21)*. The bcl-2 protein is expressed in approximately equal frequencies by neoplastic B lymphocytes in primary and secondary cutaneous follicular center cell lymphomas, suggesting that it is not a useful marker for making this distinction *(21)*. It has been suggested that bcl-2 expression in primary cutaneous large cell B cell lymphomas may be related to prognosis. Bcl-2 expression is common when these tumors occur on the legs, but not those occurring on the head and neck. These types of tumors have a much worse prognosis when they occur on the legs *(22)*.

Many other cell types in the skin express the bcl-2 oncoprotein. Basal keratinocytes weakly express this protein. Anti-bcl-2 antibodies strongly label benign and malignant melanocytes in all types of melanocytic proliferations *(23)*. A wide range of benign and malignant spindle cell tumors in the dermis also expresses the bcl-2 protein *(24)*.

TECHNICAL CONSIDERATIONS

Anti-bcl-2 antibodies that recognize antigens on routinely fixed tissue sections are commercially available. Pretreatment with enzymatic digestion or microwave antigen retrieval is essential in order to use the antibodies *(7)*. In our laboratory, we routinely pretreat with HIER in a citrate buffer to elevate the pH. This increases the sensitivity.

SUMMARY

Anti-bcl-2 has only limited utility in a diagnostic dermatopathology laboratory. The fact that bcl-2 is expressed by most circulating T cells limits one's ability to distinguish correctly bcl-2 positive B cells from T cell lymphomas in many cases. Additionally, many primary cutaneous B cell lymphomas of the follicular center cell type fail to express bcl-2, further limiting its uses. For this reason, anti-bcl-2 antibodies are not essential in diagnostic dermatopathology.

T Lymphocyte Markers
CD3

INTRODUCTION

CD3 is expressed by virtually all mature, circulating T lymphocytes. It is a surface antigen that is part of the T cell receptor complex.

DIAGNOSTIC UTILITY

Anti-CD3 is a very useful screening marker to identify cells as being T lymphocytes (Fig. 7). Unlike other pan-T cell antigens, CD3 is rarely deleted in neoplastic lymphocytes except in very undifferentiated tumors. For this reason, it is probably the best available marker to identify cells in the skin as being T lymphocytes. In the work-up of mycosis fungoides, it is helpful in serving as the marker of all T cells that can be compared with the CD4 positive and CD8 positive subsets *(25)*. It attempting to establish a diagnosis of cutaneous lymphoid hyperplasia, anti-CD3 and anti-CD20 antibodies can be used in combination to demonstrate a reactive pattern simulating nodal architecture (Fig. 8).

TECHNICAL CONSIDERATIONS

Anti-CD3 is a commercially available antibody that works very well on routinely fixed tissue sections. In most cases, enzymatic pretreatment is not necessary. However, in our laboratory, we have

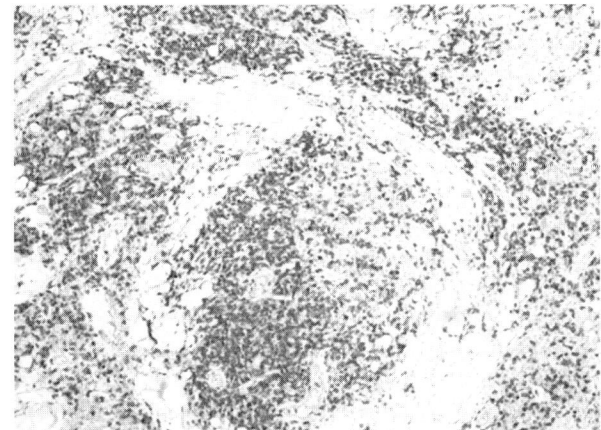

Fig. 7. CD3 expresses the majority of cells in this case of cutaneous lymphoid hyperplasia. Interspersed CD3 negative cells expressed CD20.

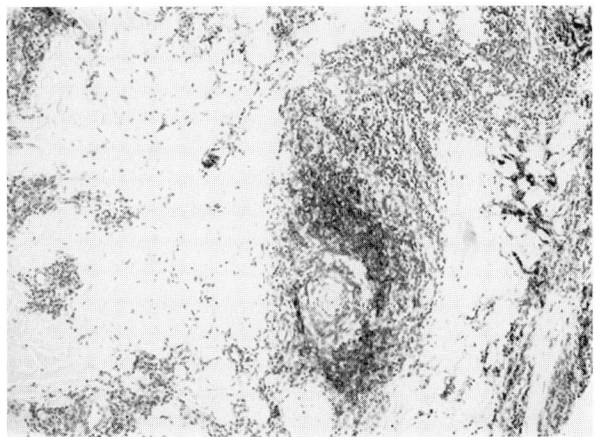

Fig. 8. CD20 staining cells in germinal centers in cutaneous lymphoid hyperplasia.

found that pretreatment with proteinase K enhances the performance of this antibody.

Summary

Anti-CD3 is an invaluable marker to be used for the identification of lymphocytes as T cells. There is essentially no cross-reactivity with any other types of hematopoietic cells and the antigen is seldom lost, even in neoplastic lymphocytes. It is an easy antibody with which to work.

CD4

INTRODUCTION

CD4 is a lymphocyte surface marker that is found on T helper lymphocytes. It is also expressed by Langerhans cells and other macrophages. In the peripheral circulation, there is normally a 4:1 ratio of CD4+ helper cells to CD8+ cytotoxic/suppressor lymphocytes. The combined use of CD4 and CD8 enables the diagnostic dermatopathologist to assess for an imbalance in this ratio. Most T cell lymphomas will demonstrate an alteration in the ratio.

DIAGNOSTIC UTILITY

Newer antibodies directed against CD4 reliably label T helper cells in formalin-fixed, paraffin-embedded tissue sections. When used in conjunction with antibodies directed against CD8, estimations of CD4/CD8 can be determined, helping in establishing a diagnosis of mycosis fungoides (Fig. 9) *(25,26)*. In B cell lymphomas, an admixture of CD4 and CD8 positive reactive T lymphocytes are present.

TECHNICAL CONSIDERATIONS

Anti-CD4 antibodies that survive formalin-fixation and paraffin embedding recently have become commercially available. The antibodies work very well in routinely processed tissue and do not require enzymatic pretreatment. In our laboratory, we have attained superior staining results with HIER pretreatment using a citrate buffer.

SUMMARY

Antibodies directed against CD4 epitopes play an essential role in the subtyping of cutaneous lymphomas. They are helpful in establishing or refuting a diagnosis of mycosis fungoides. Their use, in conjunction with anti-CD8 antibodies, is the ideal way to characterize the immunologic phenotype of dermal lymphocytic infiltrates.

CD5

INTRODUCTION

CD5 is a 67 kD glycoprotein expressed by virtually all peripheral T cells (Fig. 10). CD5 expression has also been reported on B lymphocytes in chronic lymphocytic leukemia and mantle zone lymphoma *(27)*.

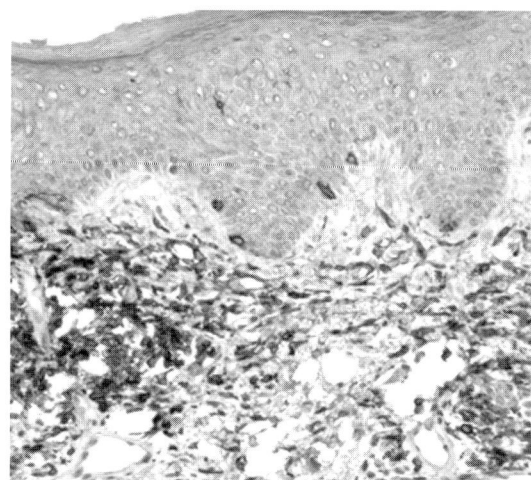

Fig. 9. CD4 stains the vast majority of cells in mycosis fungoides. CD8 is expressed by only a small minority of cutaneous T lymphocytes in this disorder (*see* Fig. 11).

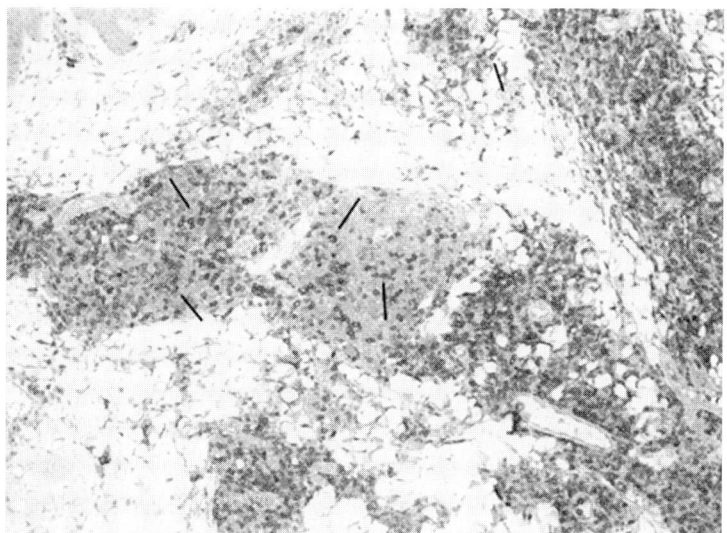

Fig. 10. CD5 is seen staining virtually all T cells within this reactive dermal infiltrate. It has only limited diagnostic utility in evaluating cutaneous lymphoid infiltrates.

DIAGNOSTIC UTILITY

The anti-CD5 antibody is useful in the work-up of cutaneous B-cell lymphomas. Cells within mantle zone lymphomas express CD5 (see Table 1). Marginal zone lymphomas and follicular center cell lymphomas do not express CD5 (28).

CD5 also labels virtually all non-Hodgkin's T cell lymphomas. While this may be helpful, it is not essential in most situations as other T cell markers provide the same information. Almost all reactive T lymphocytes express CD5 (Fig. 10).

CD5 expression is not completely specific for lymphocytes. It has also been reported on peripheral blood dendritic cells and on endothelial cells (27,29). Epithelial cells in thymic carcinomas also express CD5, but this should provide little confounding information in most cases involving the skin (30).

TECHNICAL CONSIDERATIONS

In recent years, anti-CD5 antibodies that survive routine tissue processing have become commercially available, widely increasing diagnostic utility. Microwave antigen retrieval greatly enhances signal detection when using this antibody. In our laboratory, we incubate the sections in a citrate buffer, increasing the pH. This has enhanced the staining performance of these antibodies.

SUMMARY

Anti-CD5 plays a small but definite role in diagnostic dermatopathology. It is only important to have available if the laboratory sees a significant number of cutaneous lymphomas. In these cases, it is helpful in distinguishing mantle zone lymphomas from follicular center cell and marginal zone lymphomas. As mantle zone lymphomas do not occur frequently within the skin, it may not be essential to have CD5 as a working antibody in most laboratories.

CD7

INTRODUCTION

CD7 is a 40 kD pan-T lymphocyte surface antigen that is a member of the immunoglobulin superfamily (31). It plays a role in inducing tyrosine and lipid kinase activities within the activated T lymphocyte (31). It is expressed by virtually all CD8+ T lymphocytes and greater than 90% of CD4+ cells (32). Until recently, antibodies recognizing this antigen only worked on fresh, frozen tissue. However, within the past few years, antibodies that survive routine processing have become commercially available.

Diagnostic Utility

The absence of CD7 expression has been used to provide additional evidence in favor of lymphoma. The loss of "pan-T" cell antigens such as CD7 has been reported in high grade peripheral T cell lymphomas, as well as in cases of mycosis fungoides *(33)*. However, CD7 negative T cell infiltrates have also been described in a wide range of inflammatory conditions, making this observation much less specific *(34)*.

Technical Considerations

Anti-CD7 antibodies that recognize antigens on fixed tissue specimens only recently have become available. These antibodies provide a relatively high signal to noise ratio and are fairly straightforward to use. Enzymatic pretreatment is not essential.

Summary

The use of anti-CD7 antibodies is somewhat controversial. Abundant literature suggests that CD7 expression may be decreased in cases of mycosis fungoides and that identification of a CD4+, CD8− population of cells that fail to express CD7 is strong evidence in favor of this diagnosis *(35)*. Others have refuted this observation *(36)*. With the trend toward easily available gene rearrangement studies of fixed tissue specimens, detection of CD7 expression has become less important. It may no longer be necessary to use anti-CD7 antibodies in routine diagnostic dermatopathology. Despite an extensive experience with this antibody, we no longer maintain it in our repertoire.

CD8

Introduction

CD8 is a lymphocyte surface antigen expressed by cytotoxic and suppressor T lymphocytes. These subpopulations can be further identified with more specific antibodies such as granzyme and perforin, but these have not yet gained wide acceptance in diagnostic work. For the most part, the identification of T cells as being either CD4+ helper cells or CD8+ cytotoxic/suppressor cells remains sufficient for diagnostic purposes.

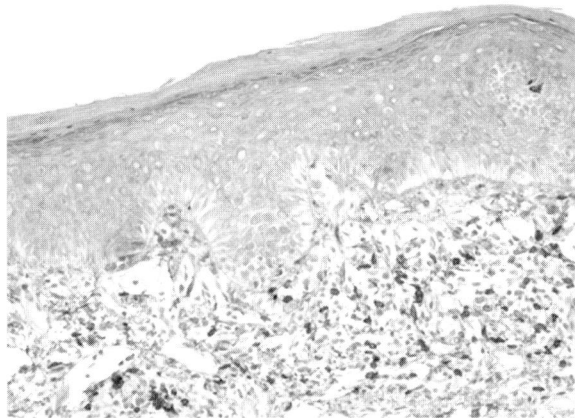

Fig. 11. CD8 labels a minority of lymphocytes present in the skin in mycosis fungoides.

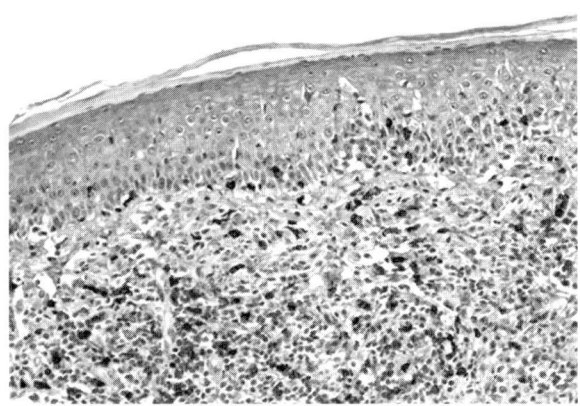

Fig. 12. Many inflammatory infiltrates demonstrate an abundance of CD8 positive lymphocytes within the epidermis.

Diagnostic Utility

Antibodies directed against CD8 are helpful in characterizing the nature of the T lymphocytes in dermal infiltrates (Fig. 11). In some conditions such as actinic reticuloid (chronic actinic dermatosis), the inflammatory infiltrate is comprised almost entirely of CD8+ cells *(37)*. In other inflammatory diseases such as lichen planus, erythema multiforme, and lichen planus, the intraepidermal components of the inflammatory process are largely CD8+ cells (Fig. 12). While precise identification of these lymphocytes is not usually necessary in order to establish these diagnoses, such immunostaining may be helpful in discriminating inflammatory dermatoses from early lesions of mycosis fungoides. Mycosis fungoides is characterized by a heavy predominance of CD4+ cells and relatively few CD8+ cells within the epidermis *(26)*. The finding of a heavily epidermotropic CD8+ infiltrate of atypical lymphocytes also may help define a rare type of epidermotropic lymphoma that in some cases is much more aggressive than is mycosis fungoides *(38)*.

TECHNICAL CONSIDERATIONS

Antibodies that recognize epitopes of the CD8 surface antigen and that survive routine tissue processing are now commercially available *(39,40)*. We have not found pretreatment with enzymes or HIER to improve the performance of these antibodies. The commercially available antibodies stain cytotoxic/suppressor lymphocytes with a very strong, clean staining pattern.

SUMMARY

Anti-CD8 antibodies are useful to have for laboratories that examine cutaneous lymphoid infiltrates. They can be very helpful in characterizing the nature of the lymphocytes within the dermis. This is useful in ruling in or out a diagnosis of mycosis fungoides or other types of cutaneous lymphomas.

CD30

INTRODUCTION

CD30 is an "activation" marker expressed on the surface of subpopulations of lymphocytes. It is a transmembrane receptor with extensive homology to tumor necrosis factor *(41)*. T cell populations that produce T helper 2 (Th2) types of cytokines preferentially express CD30 *(42)*. It was initially described on the surfaces of Reed-Sternberg cells and subsequently has been described in other conditions.

DIAGNOSTIC UTILITY

Reed-Sternberg cells in Hodgkin's disease express CD30. It is also expressed by the large, atypical cells in types A and C lymphomatoid papulosis and in large cell anaplastic lymphoma *(43,44)*. Large cell anaplastic lymphoma is currently defined as having >75% of dermal neoplastic lymphocytes expressing CD30 (Fig. 13). In lymphomatoid papulosis (type A), usually about 20–30% of cells are the large,

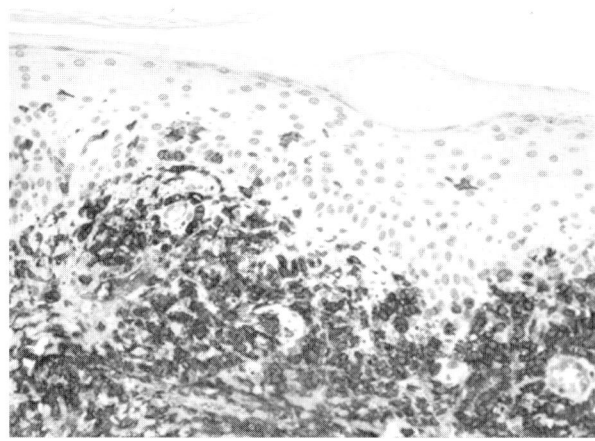

Fig. 13. CD30 labels more than 75% of atypical lymphocytes in large cell anaplastic lymphoma.

atypical cells that express CD30 (Fig. 14). Type C lymphomatoid papulosis is less well defined at this time. Some authors believe it to be closely related to or identical to primary cutaneous large cell anaplastic lymphoma. CD30 is also expressed by the cells in Burkitt's lymphomas *(44)*. Cutaneous B cell lymphomas that express CD30 have been described, but are uncommon.

Rarely, nonhematopoietic cells express CD30. The tumor cells in embryonal carcinomas label with anti-CD30 in the majority of cases. Rare cases of CD30 positive melanoma have been described *(45)*. This lack of complete specificity presents very little difficulty in differential diagnosis, however, in diagnostic dermatopathology.

TECHNICAL CONSIDERATIONS

Antibodies directed against CD30 are commercially available. These antibodies recognize epitopes that survive routine tissue processing. Tissue pretreatment with HIER is necessary in most cases *(7)*.

SUMMARY

Anti-CD30 antibodies are very helpful for the diagnostic dermatopathologist. While not common, entities such as lymphomatoid papulosis and large cell anaplastic lymphoma are largely defined by the expression of CD30 by the atypical lymphocytes. It is therefore difficult, if not impossible to make these diagnoses precisely and definitively without the antibodies.

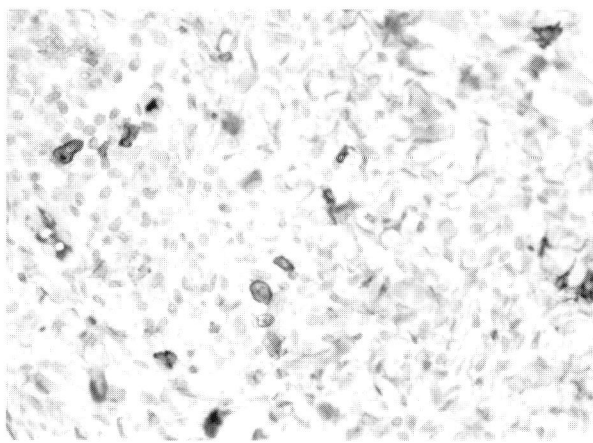

Fig. 14. CD30 recognizes a minority population of atypical lymphocytes in lymphomatoid papulosis. The majority population of small, reactive T lymphocytes fails to express CD30.

CD43

INTRODUCTION

CD43 is a pan-T lymphocyte surface marker, less commonly known as leukosialin or sialophorin *(46)*. It is an integral cell membrane mucin and appears on hematopoietic cells during embryogenesis *(47)*. It is expressed in adults in all bone marrow derived cells except in resting B lymphocytes. Thus, tissue macrophages, dendritic cells and cells in myeloid and some lymphoid leukemias express CD43 (Fig. 15). Some endothelial cells, epithelial cells, and smooth muscle cells also can express CD43 *(48)*. It is not expressed by reactive B lymphocytes, but its expression on neoplastic B lymphocytes can be used as a diagnostic clue.

DIAGNOSTIC UTILITY

One of the main uses for anti-CD43 is in the identification of B cell lymphomas (*see* Table 1). While ordinarily a T lymphocyte marker, co-expression of CD20 and CD43 occurs in a significant minority of B cell lymphomas and is associated with immunoglobulin light chain restriction (Figs. 16 and 17) *(49)*. In one study, this aberrant co-expression of CD20 and CD43 was found in 31% of small or mixed cell B cell lymphomas and in 15% of large cell lymphomas *(49)*. While rare, co-expression of CD20 and CD43 has also been reported

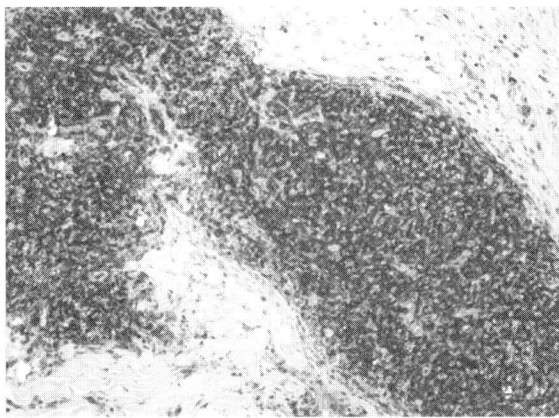

Fig. 15. A wide range of lymphoid and histiocytic cells expresses CD43.

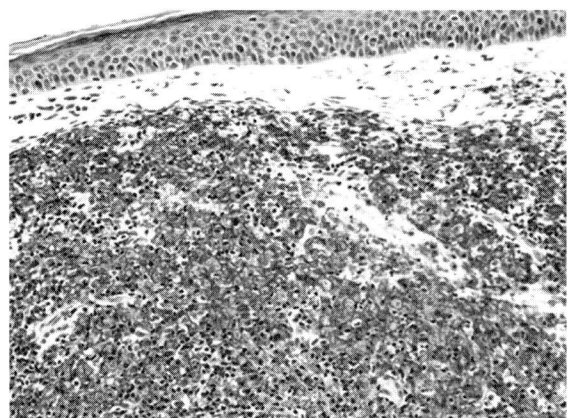

Fig. 16. CD43 is co-expressed by cells in some follicular center cell lymphomas.

in a case of infectious mononucleosis *(50)*. It is expressed in B cell lymphoma cells that also express CD5.

TECHNICAL CONSIDERATIONS

Antibodies directed against CD43 are readily available. They ordinarily do not require tissue pretreatment and work quite well in routinely fixed tissue.

SUMMARY

Anti-CD43 can be used as a marker for T lymphocytes. In this capacity, anti-CD3 antibodies that are more sensitive and do not react

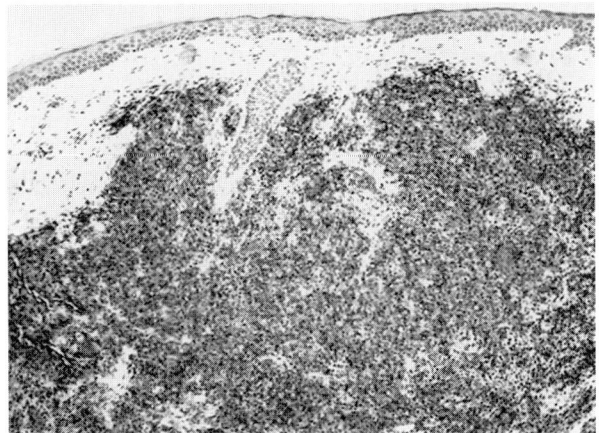

Fig. 17. The same follicular center lymphoma cells as seen in Fig. 17 also express CD20, a pan-B cell marker.

with neoplastic B lymphocytes have largely supplanted it. However, this tendency of follicular center cell neoplastic B cells to co-express CD20 and CD43 is a useful finding and very helpful diagnostically. In our laboratory, we generally reserve CD43 for this purpose, using CD3 as our first order screen for identifying T lymphocytes.

"Monocyte/Macrophage" Markers
CD1a

INTRODUCTION

CD1a is expressed, rather specifically, by cutaneous antigen presenting cells, including Langerhans cells, interdigitating and dermal dendritic cells and veiled cells *(51)*. It is a glycoprotein that plays a role in presentation of lipid antigens to T lymphocytes *(52,53)*.

DIAGNOSTIC UTILITY

CD1a expression is the most specific marker for Langerhans cells available to the diagnostic dermatopathologist. While these histiocytic cells also express HLA-DR and S100 protein, these markers are not specific. There are no other epidermotropic proliferations that express CD1a, so the finding of strong staining with this antibody in such a proliferation is diagnostic of Langerhans cell histiocytosis (Fig. 18).

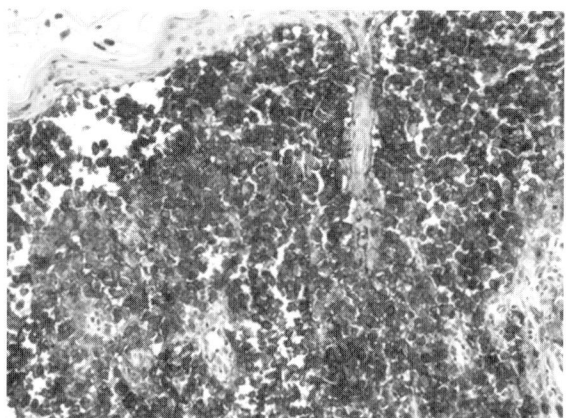

Fig. 18. Langerhans cells strongly express CD1a, as is seen in this case of Langerhans cell histiocytosis.

Interdigitating dendritic cell sarcomas are quite unusual in the skin. A minority of cases expresses CD1a *(54)*.

It is important to note that the histiocytes seen in sinus histiocytosis with massive lymphadenopathy (Rosai-Dorfman disease) fail to express CD1a. These cells share with Langerhans cells the S100 positivity, but differ in their ability to express CD1a *(55)*.

CD1a cross-reactivity with other cell types has not been reported.

TECHNICAL CONSIDERATIONS

Anti-CD1a antibodies that recognize epitopes following routine processing are available and work exceptionally well *(51,56)*. In our laboratory, HIER pretreatment has optimized our staining results.

SUMMARY

Anti-CD1a antibodies are not often needed in diagnostic dermato-pathology laboratories. However, in cases where it is necessary to establish a diagnosis of Langerhans cell histiocytosis, they are invaluable. While anti-S100 antibodies also label these cells, S100 expression is far less specific, as S100 protein is also expressed by intraepidermal melanocytes.

CD15

INTRODUCTION

CD15 is also known as sialyl Lewis X. It is a carbohydrate antigen that is present on Reed-Sternberg cells in Hodgkin's disease. It is also expressed by occasional other lymphocytes, myeloid cells and by macrophages. It is believed possibly to play a role in neutrophil adhesion by functioning as a ligand for E-selectin *(57,58)*.

DIAGNOSTIC UTILITY

Antibodies directed against CD15 are useful in confirming a diagnosis of cutaneous Hodgkin's disease. Hodgkin's disease, however, only rarely involves the skin, and in almost all cases is widely disseminated at the time of cutaneous involvement. Cells in approx 80% of cases of Hodgkin's disease express CD15. However, it should be noted that almost 20% of cases of non-Hodgkin's lymphomas had some cells that express CD15 *(59)*. Thus, while a helpful diagnostic tool, CD15 expression is not pathognomic. Rare carcinomas have been shown to express CD15 *(60)*.

TECHNICAL CONSIDERATIONS

Antibodies directed against CD15 are commercially available. They recognize epitopes of the CD15 antigen that survive routine processing. Pretreatment for antigen retrieval is usually necessary to attain maximum staining results *(7)*.

SUMMARY

There are very limited uses for anti-CD15 in diagnostic dermatopathology. It is not important to have this antibody readily available for most dermatopathology laboratories. It plays a much more central role in hematopathology laboratories.

CD68

INTRODUCTION

There are many antibodies directed against the macrophage-associated antigen CD68. CD68 is a 110 kD cytoplasmic glycoprotein and antibodies directed against several of its epitopes are available *(61)*. CD68 is a sialic acid binding lectin with relationship to the immunoglobulin superfamily *(62)*. The staining patterns of anti-CD68 antibodies differ slightly, but largely overlap. Several of these antibodies survive formalin-fixation and paraffin-embedding *(61)*. The same antigen is also present in blood neutrophils and monocytes. Some authors have suggested that CD68 is more precisely a marker of lysosomes, and not a marker for cells of the histiocytic lineage *(63)*.

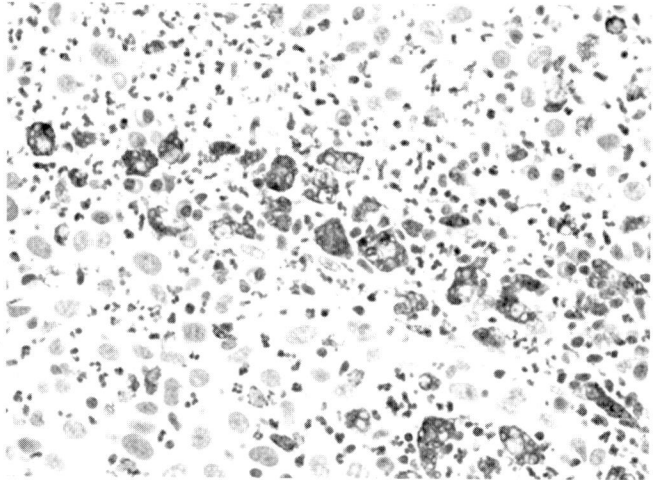

Fig. 19. Reactive dermal histiocytes express CD68.

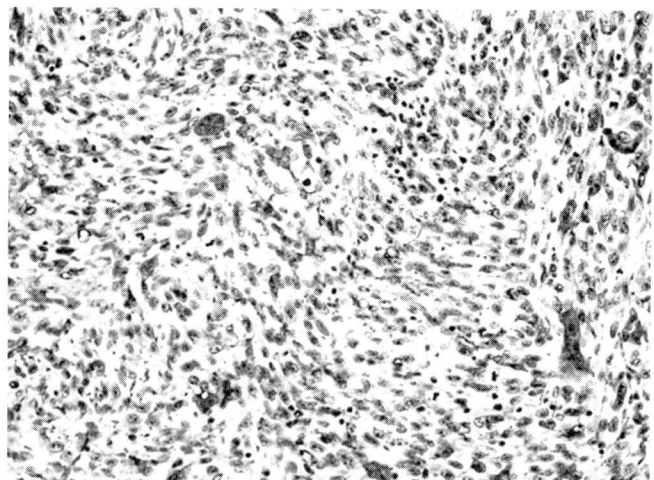

Fig. 20. A minority of cells within most atypical fibroxanthomas is seen to express CD68.

DIAGNOSTIC UTILITY

KP1, an anti-CD68 antibody, labels virutally all myeloid, myelo-monocytic and histiocytic cells (Fig. 19) *(64)*. It is valuable for establishing the diagnosis of atypical fibroxanthoma, a tumor that is positive in almost 60% of cases (Fig. 20) *(65)*. When used in conjunc-

Table 2
Essentials of Anti-CD68 Antibodies*

Types of tumors known to label with anti-CD68

Malignant fibrous histiocytoma	79%
Melanoma	70%
Renal cell carcinoma	60–100%
Large cell anaplastic lymphoma	38%
Liposarcoma	33%
Lymphomas	30%
Adenocarcinoma	25%
Malignant schwannoma	25%
Leiomyosarcoma	25%

*Antibodies work well in formalin-fixed, paraffin-embedded tissue sections.

tion with anti-actin antibodies, a diagnosis can be made with a high degree of certainty on most of these atypical spindle cell lesions. (Other antibodies are necessary to exclude tumors in the differential diagnosis, *see* Chapter 10.) It can also be used in making the diagnosis of Langerhans cell histiocytosis *(66)* though has largely been supplanted by the more specific anti-CD1a. CD68 is also somewhat helpful in establishing a diagnosis of myeloid leukemia *(67)*, but recently has been replaced with more specific markers.

Cells other than macrophages may express CD68, as is seen in Table 2. Anti-CD68 antibodies occasionally label cells in malignant melanomas, granular cells, and some neural tumors and adenocarcinomas *(68–71)*. In a large series, a minority of cells within many neoplasms was found to contain some CD68 antigen *(72)*. Mast cells react with antibodies directed against CD68 *(73)*.

TECHNICAL CONSIDERATIONS

Anti-CD68 antibodies are readily available and work well on formalin-fixed paraffin-embedded tissue sections. Pretreatment is not usually necessary to achieve staining results, though protease incubation has resulted in optimal performance in our laboratory.

SUMMARY

Anti-CD68 antibody is useful in the work-up of cutaneous lymphoid infiltrates. It serves to identify cells within an infiltrate as being histiocytic and not large lymphocytes. CD68 is also helpful in identifying the tingible body macrophages present in reactive germinal centers, but noticeably absent in neoplastic follicles. It is also helpful in the work-up of an atypical fibroxanthoma. In most other spindle cell neoplasms, CD68 is absent or only focally present, while many cells express this antigen in most atypical fibroxanthomas. However, as is seen in Table 2, a wide range of cells may express CD68, thereby greatly limiting its specificity and usefulness in establishing lineage of neoplasms *(74)*.

MAC387

Introduction

MAC387 is a monoclonal antibody that recognizes two calcium binding proteins (calgranulins) found on neutrophils and monocytes. These proteins are related to migration inhibitory factor *(75)*.

Diagnostic Utility

MAC387 is useful in identifying macrophages or histiocytes on fixed tissue sections. It also stains the cells in acute myeloid leukemia *(76)*. MAC387 has been shown to label cells within the epidermis and squamous epithelium of the cervix *(77,78)*. The significance of this observation is not known but may be related to intracellular regulation and cell proliferation.

The use of MAC387 to identify histiocytes is limited by its lack of specificity. In one study, sarcomas, the majority of adenocarcinomas, and a minority of basal cell carcinomas labeled with MAC387. In this same study, squamous cell carcinomas and melanomas did not stain *(78)*. Nonetheless, the proclivity of this antibody to label a wide range of cells limits its diagnostic utility.

Technical Considerations

The MAC387 antibody works very well on formalin-fixed, paraffin-embedded tissue sections. Pretreatment with HIER or enzymatic digestion is not ordinarily required.

Summary

The lack of specificity of this antibody precludes its routine use in diagnostic dermatopathology. For most laboratories, antibodies directed against CD68 are sufficient for identifying a population of cells as histiocytic. In very rare situations, differential expression of CD68 and the antigen recognized by MAC387 offers more precision with regard to a subset of histiocytes, but these situations are exceedingly uncommon. Thus, at this time, there is not reason to stock this antibody for most laboratories.

Other Useful Markers
Ki-67

INTRODUCTION

Ki-67 is a marker of cellular proliferation. It is a 300 kD protein present on the nuclei of cycling cells *(79)*. It is present in increasing concentrations as cells progress from G1 to S phase to mitosis. It is located within the nucleoli during G1 and in nucleoli and karyoplasm during G2 *(80)*. Ki-67 is not expressed in G0 cells. It is not specific for hematopoietic cells, but is expressed by dividing cells of all lineages.

DIAGNOSTIC UTILITY

Estimating the percentage of cells expressing Ki-67 in cutaneous lymphomas has proven to be useful in predicting outcome. When greater than 60% of B lymphocytes in a cutaneous lymphoma express Ki-67, survival is significantly decreased *(33)*. It has been suggested that using Ki-67 to assess a proliferation index may provide some useful prognostic information, especially in lymphoproliferative processes *(81)*. It also may provide useful prognostic information for breast and prostate cancers, and melanomas *(79,82)*.

Investigators have used Ki-67 staining in attempt to differentiate melanomas from various types of benign melanocytic proliferations. While this technique has met with some degree of success *(83,84)*, there is extensive overlap in the observed results *(85)*. This has prevented this type of analysis from widespread use as a diagnostic test.

TECHNICAL CONSIDERATIONS

Antibodies directed against Ki-67 recognize epitopes that are stable with routine processesing. They are easy to work with and provide a good signal to noise ratio without tissue pretreatment. HIER has been shown to augment the staining intensity *(7)*.

SUMMARY

Ki-67 antibodies play a small role in diagnostic dermatopathology. This role is still evolving. Certainly, elevated rates of Ki-67 positive lymphocytes favor a lymphoma over a reactive process.

However, some Ki-67 positive lymphocytes are present in all reactive inflammatory infiltrates. Ki-67 positive melanocytes are seen more commonly in melanomas than in benign nevoid proliferations. However, these data are still be evaluated and are still not particularly helpful in a case by case basis.

CD56

INTRODUCTION

CD56 is also known as neuronal cell adhesion marker (NCAM) *(86)*. It is expressed on the surface of natural killer cells as well as on neural tissues.

DIAGNOSTIC UTILITY

Antibodies directed against CD56 are helpful in establishing a diagnosis of natural killer cell lymphomas in the skin *(87)*. It is useful to add this marker to the work-up of a dense, angiodestructive lymphoid infiltrate in attempting to make a diagnosis of a NK lymphoma *(86)*. Another marker of NK cells, CD57, is frequently negative in these cutaneous lymphomas *(88–90)*. Acute leukemias can also express CD56 *(88)*. These antibodies can also be used in establishing the neural origin of tumors such as neurofibromas, and myxoid neurothekeomas (*see* Chapter 7).

TECHNICAL CONSIDERATIONS

Anti-CD56 antibodies are highly sensitive and specific for natural killer cells. Less than 0.1% of cells within the normal dermal inflammatory infiltrate express this marker. Rare plasma cells may demonstrate cytoplasmic staining with the antibodies *(87)*.

SUMMARY

Antibodies directed against CD56 are not essential in diagnostic dermatopathology. They can be helpful in the complete work-up of some angiocentric lymphomas. However, these are quite rare. For this reason, most laboratories have little use for this marker. We have found this antibody to be invaluable in exceptional cases.

Mast Cell Tryptase
Introduction

Mast cell tryptase is a cytoplasmic serine protease relatively specific for mast cells *(91)*.

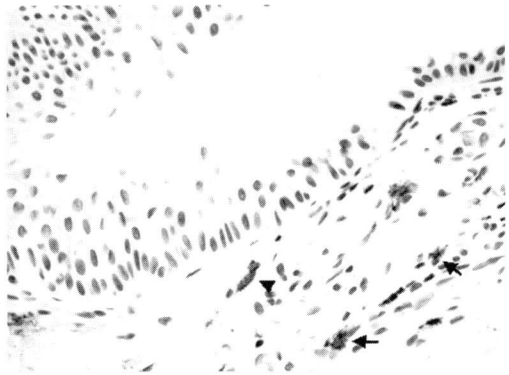

Fig. 21. Mast cell tryptase is a sensitive and specific method for detecting cutaneous mast cells.

Diagnostic Utility

Antibodies directed against mast cell tryptase were found to be 100% sensitive for mast cells in one large study. In this study, these antibodies were significantly more sensitive in detecting mast cells than were giemsa or chloroacetate esterase stains *(91)*. The antibody has also been shown to be very specific for mast cells, not staining other cells with cytoplasmic granules such as myeloid precursors (Fig. 21) *(92)*.

Technical Considerations

Antibodies directed against mast cell tryptase recognize epitopes that survive routine processing. They provide strong, granular cytoplasmic staining and do not require pretreatment with enzymes or HIER. However, in our laboratory, we have found that pretreatment with protease enhances the staining sensitivity.

Summary

There is not yet an extensive literature concerning these antibodies that only recently have been described. Nonetheless, the published literature suggests that use of these antibodies may be a more sensitive and specific method for detecting mast cells in routinely processed tissue than is the performance of routine histochemical stains. We have had the same experience and now use anti-mast cell tryptase antibodies in place of giemsa, toluidine blue, or chloroacetate esterase stains.

CD99

CD99 is discussed in Chapter 7.

References

1. Kurtin, P. J. and Pinkus, G. S. (1985) Leukocyte common antigen—a diagnostic discriminant between hematopoietic and nonhematopoietic neoplasms in paraffin sections using monoclonal antibodies: correlation with immunologic studies and ultrastructural localization. *Hum. Pathol.* **16,** 353–365.
2. Fischer, E. H., Charbonneau, H., Cool, D. E., and Tonks, N. K. (1992) Tyrosine phosphatases and their possible interplay with tyrosine kinases. *Ciba Found. Symp.* **164,** 132–140.
3. Clark, E. A. and Ledbetter, J. A. (1989) Leukocyte cell surface enzymology CD45 (LCA, T200) is a protein tyrosine phosphatase. *Immunol. Today* **10,** 225–228.
4. Clement, L. T. (1992) Isoforms of the CD45 common leukocyte antigen family: markers for human T-cell differentiation. *J. Clin. Immunol.* **12,** 1–10.
5. Burg, G., Kerl, H., Kaudewitz, P., Braun-Falco, O., and Mason, D. Y. (1984) Immunoenzymatic typing of lymphoplasmacytoid skin infiltrates. *J. Dermatol. Surg. Oncol.* **10,** 284–290.
6. Baldassano, M. F., Bailey, E. M., Ferry, J. A., Harris, N. L., and Duncan, L. M. (1999) Cutaneous lymphoid hyperplasia and cutaneous marginal zone lymphoma: comparison of morphologic and immunophenotypic features. *Am. J. Surg. Pathol.* **23,** 88–96.
7. Gown, A. M., de Wever, N., and Battifora, H. (1993) Microwave-based antigenic unmasking. A revolutionary new technique for routine immunohistochemistry. *Appl. Immunohistochem.* **1,** 256–266.
8. Bene, M. C. and Faure, G. C. (1997) CD10 in acute leukemias, GEIL (Groupe d'etude immunologique des leucemies). *Haematologica* **82,** 205–210.
9. Franco, R., Fernandez-Vasquez, A., Rodriguez-Peralto, J. L., Bellas, C., Lopez-Rios, F., Saez, A., Villuendas, R., Navarrete, M., Fernandez, I., Zarco, C., and Piris, M. A. (2001) Cutaneous follicular B-cell lymphoma: description of a series of 18 cases. *Am. J. Surg. Pathol.* **25,** 875–883.
10. Freedman, A. S. and Nadler, L. M. (1991) Immunologic markers in non-Hodgkin's lymphoma. *Hematol. Oncol. Clin. North Am.* **5,** 871–889.
11. Kurtin, P. J. (1998) Mantle zone lymphoma. *Adv. Anat. Pathol.* **5,** 376–398.
12. Pimpinelli, N. and Santucci, M. (2000) The skin-associated lymphoid tissue-related B-cell lymphomas. *Semin. Cutan. Med. Surg.* **19,** 124–129.
13. Carrel, S., Zografos, L., Schereyer, M., and Rimoldi, D. (1993) Expression of CALLA/CD10 on human melanoma cells. *Melanoma Res.* **3,** 19–23.
14. Beljaards, R. C., Meijer, C. J., Scheffer, E., van der Valk, P., and Willemze, R. (1991) Differential diagnosis of cutaneous large cell lymphomas using monoclonal antibodies reactive in paraffin-embedded skin biopsy specimens. *Am. J. Dermatopathol.* **13,** 342–349.
15. Tedder, T. F. and Engel, P. (1994) CD20: a regulator of cell-cycle progression of B lymphocytes. *Immunol. Today* **15,** 450–454.
16. Toyota, N., Matsuo, S., and Iizuka, H. (1991) Immunohistochemical differential diagnosis between lymphocytoma cutis and malignant lymphoma in paraffin-embedded sections. *J. Dermatol.* **18,** 586–591.

17. Nagatani, T., Miyazawa, M., Matsuzaki, T., Hayakawa, H., Iemoto, G., Kim, S. T., et al. (1993) Cutaneous B cell lymphoma—a clinical, pathological and immunohistochemical study. *Clin. Exp. Dermatol.* **18**, 530–536.

18. Chu, P. G. and Arber, D. A. (2001) CD79: a review. Appl. Immunohistochem. *Molecul. Morphol.* **9**, 97–106.

19. Troussard, X., Maloisel, F., and Flandrin, G. (1998) Hairy cell leukemia. What is new forty years after the first description? *Hematol. Cell. Ther.* **40**, 139–148.

20. LeBrun, D. E., Warnke, R. A., and Clearly, M. L. (1993) Expression of bcl-2 in fetal tissues suggests a role in morphogenesis. *Am. J. Pathol.* **142**, 745–753.

21. Triscott, J. A., Ritter, J. H., Swanson, P. E., and Wick, M. R. (1995) Immunoreactivity for bcl-2 protein in cutaneous lymphomas and lymphoid hyperplasias. *J. Cutan. Pathol.* **22**, 2–10.

22. Geelen, F. A., Vermeer, M. H., Meijer, C. J., Van der Putte, S. C., Kerkhof, E., Kluin, P. M., and Willemze, R. (1998) bcl-2 protein expression in primary cutaneous large B-cell lymphoma is site-related. *J. Clin. Oncol.* **16**, 2080–2085.

23. Morales-Ducret, J., van de Rijn, M., and Smoller, B. R. (1995) bcl-2 expression in melanocytic nevi. Insights into the biology of dermal maturation. *Arch. Dermatol.* **131**, 915–918.

24. Suster, S., Fisher, C., and Moran, C. A. (1998) Expression of bcl-2 oncoprotein in benign and malignant spindle cell tumors of soft tissue, skin, serosal surfaces, and gastrointestinal tract. *Am. J. Surg. Pathol.* **22**, 863–872.

25. Izban, K. F., Hsi, E. D., and Alkan, S. (1998) Immunohistochemical analysis of mycosis fungoides on paraffin-embedded tissue sections. *Mod. Pathol.* **11**, 978–982.

26. Nuckols, J. D., Shea, C. R., Horenstein, M. G., Burchette, J. L., and Prieto, V. (1999) Quantitation of intraepidermal T-cell subsets in formalin-fixed, paraffin-embedded tissue helps in the diagnosis of mycosis fungoides. *J. Cutan. Pathol.* **26**, 169–175.

27. Arber, D. A. and Weiss, L. (1995) CD5: a review. *Appl. Immunohistochem.* **3**, 1–22.

28. Dorfman, D. M. and Shahsafaei, M. S. (1997) Usefulness of a new CD5 antibody for the diagnosis of T-cell and B-cell lymphoproliferative disorders in paraffin sections. *Mod. Pathol.* **10**, 859–863.

29. Gogolin-Ewens, K., Meeusen, E., Lee, C. S., and Brandon, M. (1989) Expression of CD5, a lymphocyte surface antigen on the endothelium of blood vessels. *Eur. J. Immunol.* **19**, 935–938.

30. Dorfman, D. M., Shahsafaei, M. S., and Chan, J. K. C. (1997) Thymic carcinomas, but not thymomas and carcinoma of other sites, show CD5 immunoreactivity. *Am. J. Surg. Pathol.* **21**, 936–940.

31. Stillwell, R. and Bierer, B. E. (2001) T cell signal transduction and the role of CD7 in costimulation. *Immunol. Res.* **24**, 31–52.

32. Reinhold, U., Abken, H., Kukel, S., Moll, M., Muller, R., Oltermann, I., and Kreysel, H. W. (1993) CD7- T cells represent a subset of normal human blood lymphocytes. *J. Immunol.* **150**, 2081–2089.

33. Chott, A., Augustin, I., Wrba, F., Hanak, H., Ohlinger, W., and Radaszkiewicz, T. (1990) Peripheral T-cell lymphomas: a clinicopatohlogic study of 75 cases. *Hum. Pathol.* **21**, 1117–1125.

34. Smoller, B. R., Bishop, K., Glusac, E. J., Kim, Y. H., Bhargava, V., and Warnke, R. A. (1995) Lymphocyte antigen abnormalities in inflammatory dermatoses. *Appl. Immunohistochem.* **3**, 127–131.

35. Wood, G. S., Abel, E. A., Hoppe, R. T., and Warnke, R. A. (1986) Leu-8 and leu-9 antigen phenotypes: immunologic criteria for the distinction of mycosis fungoides drom cutaneous inflammation. *J. Am. Acad. Dermatol.* **14,** 1006–1013.

36. Ralfkiaer, E., Wantzin, G. L., Mason, D. Y., Hou-Jensen, K., Stein, H., and Thomsen, K. (1985) Phenotypic characterization of lymphocyte subsets in mycosis fungoides: comparison with large plaque parapsoriasis and benign chronic dermatoses. *Am. J. Clin. Pathol.* **84,** 610–619.

37. Toonstra, J. (1991) Actinic reticuloid. *Semin. Diagn. Pathol.* **8,** 109–116.

38. Quarterman, M. J., Lesher, J. L., Jr., Davis, L. S., Pantazis, C. G., and Mullins, S. (1995) Rapidly progressive CD-positive cutaneous T-cell lymphoma with tongue involvement. *Am. J. Dermatopathol.* **17,** 287–291.

39. Mason, D. Y., Cordell, J. L., Gaulard, P., Tse, A. G., and Brown, M. H. (1992) Immunohistochemical detection of human cytotoxic/supressor T cells using antibodies to a CD8 peptide sequence. *J. Clin. Pathol.* **45,** 1084–1088.

40. Williamson, S. L., Steward, M., Milton, I., Parr, A., Piggott, N. H., Krajewski, A. S., Angus, B., and Horne, C. H. (1998) New monoclonal antibodies to the T cell antigens CD4 and CD8. Production and characterization in formalin-fixed paraffin-embedded tissue. *Am. J. Pathol.* **152,** 1421–1426.

41. de Bruin, P. C., Gruss, H. J., van der Valk, P., Willemze, R., and Meijer, C. J. (1995) CD30 expression in normal and neoplastic lymphoid tissue: biological aspects and clinical implications. *Leukemia* **9,** 1620–1627.

42. Del Prete, G., Maggi, E., Pizzolo, G., and Raomagnani, S. (1995) CD30, Th2 cytokines and HIV infectoin: a complex and fascinating link. *Immunol. Today* **16,** 76–80.

43. Cerroni, L., Smolle, J., Soyer, H. P., Martinez Aparicio, A., and Kerl, H. (1990) Immunophenotyping of cutaneous lymphoid infiltrates in frozen and paraffin-embedded tissue sections: a comparative study. *J. Am. Acad. Dermatol.* **22,** 405–413.

44. Gruss, H. J. and Herrmann, F. (1996) CD30 ligand, a member of the TNF ligand superfamily, with growth and activation control CD30+ lymphoid and lymphoma cells. *Leuk. Lymphoma* **20,** 397–406.

45. Polski, J. M. and Janney, C. G. (1999) Ber-H2 (CD30) immunohistochemical staining in malignant melanoma. *Mod. Pathol.* **12,** 903–906.

46. Fukuda, M. (1991) Leukosialin, a major O-glycan-containing sialoglycoprotein defining leukocyte differentiation and malignancy. *Glycobiology* **1,** 347–356.

47. Rosenstein, Y., Santana, A., and Pedraza-Alva, G. (1999) CD43, a molecule with multiple functions. *Immunol. Res.* **20,** 89–99.

48. Rupniewska, Z. M., Rolinski, J., and Bojarska-Junak, A. (2000) Universal CD43 molecule. *Postepy Hig. Med. Dosw.* **54,** 619–638.

49. Ritter, J. H., Adesokan, P. N., Fitzgibbon, J. F., and Wick, M. R. (1994) Paraffin section immunohistochemistry as an adjunct to morphologic analysis in the diagnosis of cutaneous lymphoid infiltrates. *J. Cutan. Pathol.* **21,** 481–493.

50. Shin, S. S., Berry, G. J., and Weiss, L. M. (1991) Infectious mononucleosis: Diagnosis by in situ hybridization in two cases with atypical features. *Am. J. Surg. Pathol.* **15,** 625–631.

51. Krenacs, L., Tiszalvicz, L., Krenacs, T., and Boumsell, L. (1993) Immunohistochemical detection of CD1A antigen in formalin-fixed and paraffin-embedded tissue sections with monoclonal antibody O10. *J. Pathol.* **171,** 99–104.

52. Chu, T. and Jaffe, R. (1994) The normal Langerhans cell and the LCH cell. *Brit. J. Cancer Suppl.* **23,** S4–10.

53. Moody, D. B., Besra, G. S., Wilson, I. A., and Porcelli, S. A. (1999) The molecular basis of CD1-mediated presentation of lipid antigens. *Immunol. Rev.* **172,** 285–296.
54. Gaertner, E. M., Tsokos, M., Derringer, G. A., Neuhauser, T. S., Arciero, C., and Andriko, J. A. (2001) Interdigitating dendritic cell sarcoma. A report of four cases and review of the literature. *Am. J. Clin. Pathol.* **115,** 589–597.
55. Lu, D., Estalilla, O. C., Manning, J. T., Jr., and Medeiros, L. J. (2000) Sinus histiocytosis with massive lymphadenopathy and malignant lymphoma involving the same lymph node: a report of four cases and review of the literature. *Mod. Pathol.* **13,** 414–419.
56. Emile, J. F., Weschler, J., Brousse, N., Boulland, M. L., Cologon, R., Fraitag, S., et al. (1995) Langerhans' cell histiocytesis. Definitive diagnosis with the use of monoclonal antibody O10 on routinely paraffin-embedded samples. *Am. J. Surg. Pathol.* **19,** 636–641.
57. Kerr, M. A. and Stocks, S. C. (1992) The role of CD15-(Le(X))-related carbohydrates in neutrophil adhesion. *Histochem.* **24,** 811–826.
58. Kannagi, R. (1997) Carbohydrate-mediated cell adhesion involved in hematogenous metastsis of cancer. *Gylcoconj. J.* **14,** 577–584.
59. Hall, P. A. and D'Ardenne, A. J. (1987) Value of CD15 immunostaining in diagnosis Hodgkin's disease: a review of published literature. *J. Clin. Pathol.* **40,** 1298–1304.
60. Kornstein, M. J., Bonner, H., Gee, B., Cohen, R., and Brooks, J. J. (1986) Leu M1 and S100 in Hodgkin's disease and non-Hodgkin's lymphomas. *Am. J. Clin. Pathol.* **85,** 433–437.
61. Saito, N., Pulford, K. A., Breton-Gorius, J., Masse, J. M., Mason, D. Y., and Cramer, E. M. (1991) Ultrastructural localization of CD68 macrophage-associated antigen in human blood neutrophils and monocytes. *Am. J. Pathol.* **139,** 1053–1059.
62. Martinez-Pomares, L., Platt, N., McKnight, A. J., da Silva, R. P., and Gordon, S. (1996) Macrophage membrane molecules: markers of tissue differentiation and heterogeneity. *Immunobiology* **195,** 407–416.
63. Tsang, W. Y. and Chan, J. K. C. (1992) KP1 (CD68) staining of granular cell neoplasms: is KP1 a marker for lysosomes rather than the histiocytic lineage? *Histopathology* **21,** 84–86.
64. Warnke, R. A., Pulford, K. A., Pallesen, G., Ralfkaier, E., Brown, D. C., Gatter, K. C., and Mason, D. Y. (1989) Diagnosis of myelomonocytic and macrophage neoplasms in routinely processed tissue biopsies with monoclonal antibody KP1. *Am. J. Pathol.* **135,** 1089–1095.
65. Longacre, T. A., Smoller, B. R., and Rouse, R. V. (1993) Atypical fibro-xanthoma. Multiple immunohistologic profiles. *Am. J. Surg. Pathol.* **17,** 1199–1209.
66. Ornvold, K., Ralfkaier, E., and Carstensen, H. (1990) Immunohistochemical study of the abnormal cells in Langerhans cell histiocytosis (histiocytosis X). *Virchows Arch. A Pathol. Anat. Histopathol.* **416,** 403–410.
67. Davey, F. R., Elghetany, M. T., and Kurec, A. S. (1990) Immunophenotyping of hematologic neoplasms in paraffin-embedded tissue sections. *Am. J. Clin. Pathol.* **93, 4 suppl 1,** S17–26.
68. Facchetti, F., Bertalot, G., and Grigolato, P. G. (1991) KP1 (CD68) staining of malignant melanomas. *Histopathology* **19,** 141–145.
69. De i Tos, A. P., Doglioni, C., Laurino, L., and Fletcher, C. D. M. (1993) KP1 (CD68) experssion in benign neural tumours. Further evidence of its low specificity as a histiocytic/myeloid marker. *Histopathology* **23,** 185–187.
70. Kaiserling, E., Xaio, J. C., Ruck, P., and Horny, H. P. (1993) Aberrant expression of macrophage-associated antigens (CD68 and Ki-M1P) by Schwann cells

in reactive and neoplastic neural tissue. Light- and electorn-microscopic findings. *Mod. Pathol.* **6,** 463–468.

71. Doussis, I. A., Gatter, K. C., and Mason, D. Y. (1993) CD68 reactivity of non-macrophage derived tumours in cytological specimens. *J. Clin. Pathol.* **46,** 334–336.

72. Gloghini, A., Rizzo, A., Zanette, I., Canal, B., Rupolo, G., Bassi, P., and Carbone, A. (1995) KP1/CD68 expression in malignant neoplasms including lymphomas, sarcomas, and carcinomas. *Am. J. Clin. Pathol.* **103,** 425–431.

73. Horny, H. P., Schaumburg-Lever, G., Bolz, S., Geerts, M. L., and Kaiserling, E. (1990) Use of monoclonal antibody KP1 for identifying normal and neoplastic human mast cells. *J. Clin. Pathol.* **43,** 89–90.

74. Cassidy, M., Loftus, B., Whelan, A., Sabt, B., Hickey, D., Henry, K., and Leader, M. (1994) KP-1: not a specific marker. Staining of 137 sarcomas, 48 lymphomas, 28 carcinomas, 7 malignant melanomas and 8 cystosarcoma phyllodes. *Virchows Arch.* **424,** 635–640.

75. Chilosi, M., Mombello, A., Montagna, L., Benedetti, A., Lestani, M., Semenzato, G., and Menestrina, F. (1990) Multimarker immunohistochemical staining of calgranulins, chloroacetate esterase, and S100 for simultaneous demonstration of inflammatory cells on paraffin sections. *J. Histochem. Cytochem.* **38,** 1669–1675.

76. Horny, H. P., Campbell, M., Steinke, B., and Kaiserling, E. (1990) Acute myeloid leukemia: immunohistologic findings in paraffin-embedded bone marrow biopsy specimens. *Hum. Pathol.* **21,** 648–655.

77. Coleman, N. and Stanley, M. A. (1994) Expression of the myelomonocytic antigens CD36 and L1 by keratinocytes in squamous intraepithelial lesions of the cervix. *Hum. Pathol.* **25,** 73–79.

78. Loftus, B., Loh, L. C., Curran, B., Henry, K., and Leader, M. (1991) Mac387: its non-specificity as a tumour marker or marker of histiocytes. *Histopathology* **19,** 251–255.

79. Gerdes, J. (1990) Ki-67 and other proliferation markers useful for immunohistological diagnostic and prognostic evaluations in human malignancies. *Semin. Cancer Biol.* **1,** 199–206.

80. Sieigneurin, D. and Guillaud, P. (1991) Ki-67 antigen, a cell cycle and tumor growth marker. *Pathol. Biol. (Paris)* **39,** 1020–1028.

81. Brown, D. C. and Gatter, K. C. (1990) Monoclonal antibody Ki-67: its use in histopathology. *Histopathology* **17,** 489–503.

82. Scholzen, T. and Gerdes, J. (2000) The Ki-67 protein: from the known and the unknown. *J. Cell. Physiol.* **182,** 311–322.

83. Li, L. X., Crotty, K. A., McCarthy, S. W., Palmer, A. A., and Kril, J. J. (2000) A zonal comparison of MIB1-Ki67 immunoreactivity in benign and malignant melanocytic lesions. *Am. J. Dermatopathol.* **22,** 489–495.

84. Bergman, R., Malkin, L., Sabo, E., and Kerner, H. (2001) MIB-1 monoclonal antibody to determine proliferative activity of Ki-67 antigen as an adjunct to the histopathologic differential diagnosis of Spitz nevi. *J. Am. Acad. Dermatol.* **44,** 500–504.

85. McNutt, N. S., Urmacher, C., Hakimian, J., Hoss, D. M., and Lugo, J. (1995) Nevoid malignant melanoma: morphologic patterns and immunohistochemical reactivity. *J. Cutan. Pathol.* **22,** 502–517.

86. Wong, K. F., Chan, J. K., and Ng, C. S. (1994) CD56 (NCAM)-positive malignant lymphoma. *Leuk. Lymphoma* **14,** 29–36.

87. Tsang, W. Y., Chan, J. K., Ng, C. S., and Pau, M. Y. (1996) Utility of a paraffin section-reactive CD56 antibody (123C3) for characterization and diagnosis of lymphomas. *Am. J. Surg. Pathol.* **20,** 202–210.

88. Suzuki, R. and Nakamura, S. (1999) Malignancies of natural killer (NK) cell precursor: myeloid/NK cell precursor acute leukemia and blastic NK cell lymphoma/ leukemia. *Leuk. Res.* **23,** 615–624.

89. Chan, J. K., Sin, V. C., Wong, K. F., Ng, C. S., Tsang, W. Y., Chan, C. H., et al. (1997) Nonnasal lymphoma expressing the natural killer cell marker CD56: a clinicopathologic study of 49 csaes of an uncommon aggressive neoplasm. *Blood* **89,** 4501–4513.

90. Weiss, L. M., Arber, D. A., and Strickler, J. G. (1994) Nasal T-cell lymphoma. *Ann. Oncol.* **5 suppl 1,** 39–42.

91. Horny, H. P., Sillaber, C., Menke, D., Kaiserling, E., Wehrmann, M., Stehberger, B., et al. (1998) Diagnostic value of immunostaining for tryptase in patients with mastocytosis. *Am. J. Surg. Pathol.* **22,** 1132–1140.

92. Li, W. V., Kapadia, S. B., Sonmez-Alpan, E., and Swerdlow, S. H. (1996) Immunohistochemical characterization of mast cell disease in paraffin sections using tryptase, CD68, myeloperoxidase, lysozyme, and CD20 antibodies. *Mod. Pathol.* **9,** 982–988.

6 Melanocyte Markers

S100 Protein

Introduction

Antibodies directed against S100 protein were the first widely available markers used in the identification of melanocytes. S100 protein was initially detected within the brain in 1965 *(1)*. It is a thermolabile protein, and functions as an acidic calcium-binding protein. The protein is composed of α and β subunits. Langerhans cells contain exclusively the β subunit of S100, while melanocytes contain α and β subunits *(2)*. Macrophages solely express the α subunit of the S100 protein in most circumstances. Neutrophils and adipocytes within the subcutaneous fat also express S100 protein *(3)*.

Diagnostic Utility

Despite its lack of total specificity, antibodies directed against S100 protein continue to play a central role in establishing a diagnosis of melanoma in the skin. The routinely used, commercially available polyclonal antibodies are directed against both subunits of S100 protein and recognize proteins expressed in melanocytes, Langerhans cells, neutrophils, and nerves within the skin. In some settings, macrophages may also be detected with anti-S100 protein antibodies. It is important to note that virtually all melanocytes, whether occurring singly in the epidermis, as benign nevus nests, or as melanoma cells, express S100 protein within their cytoplasms (Figs. 1 and 2). Reported sensitivity rates for melanoma range from 83–100% *(4,5)*. Similar high sensitivity rates have been reported for less common subtypes including mucosal, sinonasal and desmoplastic melanomas *(6,7)*. Metastatic melanoma is also almost always detected with anti-S100 protein antibodies (Table 1). Melanomas may fail to express S100 protein, though this is exceedingly uncommon *(8)*.

When attempting to identify a subpopulation of cells within the epidermis, it is important to evaluate the immunostaining in concert

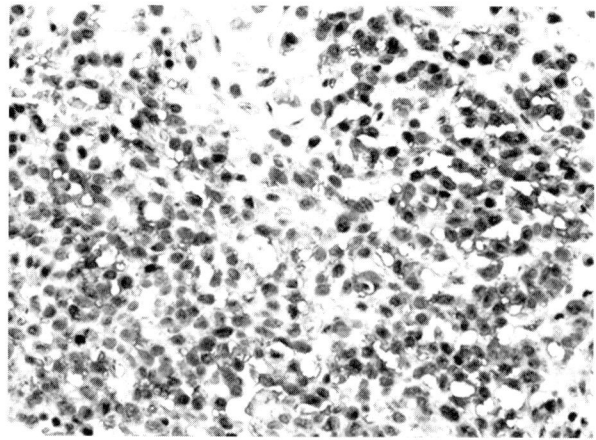

Fig. 1. Strong staining of all nevus cells with anti-S100 protein antibody is seen in most benign melanocytic nevi.

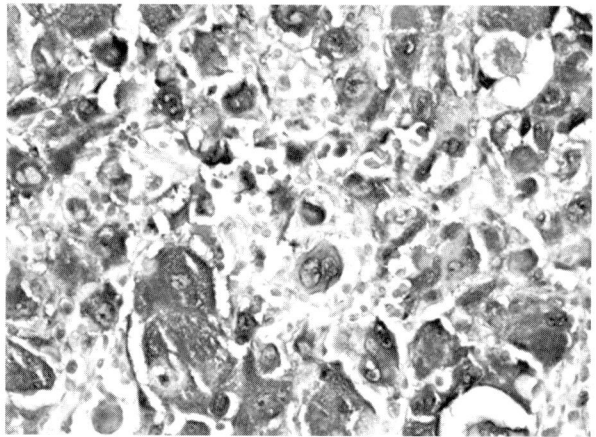

Fig. 2. Similar strong, diffuse staining with anti-S100 protein antibody is seen within the cells of most melanomas.

with the routine histology in order to separate Langerhans cells from melanocytes (Fig. 3). (The addition of an anti-CD1a antibody would further help in this distinction, as Langerhans cells invariably express this antigen, while melanocytes do not). More commonly, dermato-pathologists are asked to identify a population of poorly differenti-ated spindle-shaped cells within the dermis. In this setting, anti-S100 protein antibodies can be an invaluable aid. Virtually all desmoplas-

Table 1
Anti-S100 Protein Antibody Essentials*

Melanocytic proliferations	Sensitivity
Primary cutaneous melanoma	83–100%
Desmoplastic melanoma	<100%
Mucosal melanoma	<100%
Sinonasal melanoma	<100%
Metastatic melanoma	<100%
Common acquired melanocytic nevi	<100%
Spitz nevi	<100%
Dysplastic nevi	<100%

Other known positively staining tumors

Rosai-Dorfman disease
Chordoma
Parachordoma
Langerhans cell histiocytoses
Ossifying fibromyxoid tumor of soft parts
Chondrosarcoma
Neurofibroma
Schwannoma
Granular cell tumor
Myxoid neurothekeoma
Clear cell sarcoma
Malignant peripheral nerve sheath tumor
Neuromuscular choristoma
Rhabdomyosarcoma
Liposarcomas
Syringoma
Mixed tumors of the skin
Breast carcinoma
Salivary gland tumors
Lung carcinomas

*Paraffin-embedded, formalin-fixed tissue, pretreatment with trypsin necessary for monoclonal antibodies with some manufacturers, no pretreatment necessary for polyclonal antibody, cytoplasmic and nuclear staining.

tic melanomas express this protein, and virtually none of the other neoplasms in this histologic differential diagnosis do so. Thus, results from this test are very helpful in narrowing a differential diagnosis, and when used in conjunction with other antibodies, can help establish a diagnosis in most cases (*see* Chapter 10).

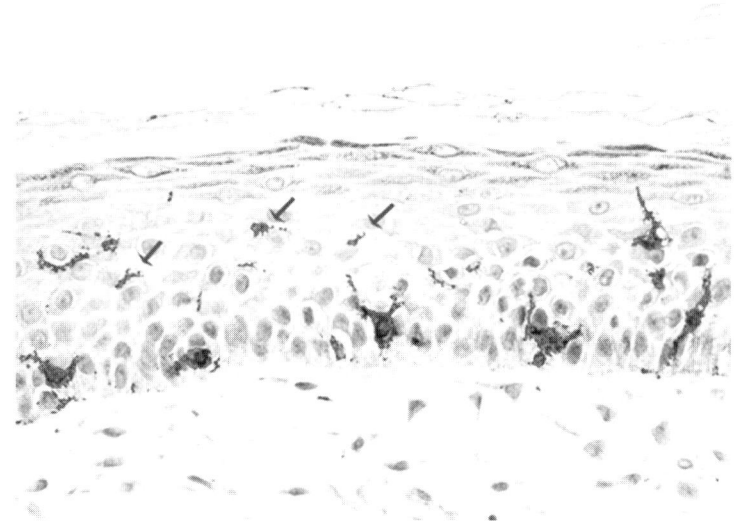

Fig. 3. Intraepidermal Langerhans cells and melanocytes both express S100 protein. Arrows represent Langerhans cells expressing S100 protein.

Technical Considerations

The original antibodies developed against the S100 protein were polyclonal and identified both subunits of the protein. Newer antibodies are monoclonal and may be directed against the specific α or β subunits. All of these antibodies work well on formalin-fixed, paraffin-embedded tissue. Some of the monoclonal antibodies require tissue trypsinization prior to immunostaining, depending upon the manufacturer *(8)*. These antibodies can help to identify cells of origin based upon differential expression of α or β subunits, but have not yet gained commonplace usage in the clinical laboratories. Nerves and melanocytes normally present in the skin serve as positive internal controls for evaluating the adequacy of the staining procedure. Nuclear and cytoplasmic stains are seen with anti-S100 antibodies. HIER may be helpful in increasing the intensity of staining with the polyclonal anti-S100 antibody *(9)*.

Summary

Anti -S100 protein antibodies detect benign and malignant melanocytes and are thus of no use in determining the biologic behavior of a melanocytic proliferation. If the cell type giving rise to the proliferation cannot be ascertained using routine histologic sections, anti-S100 can be invaluable in distinguishing melanocytes from other potential cell types. This is especially true for primary cutaneous neoplasms, given the limited numbers of cell types normally present in the skin that will express this protein (Table 1). Anti-S100 antibodies are also useful as a screening measure when examining sentinel lymph nodes for the presence of metastatic melanoma. The presence of individually staining cells should be interpreted with extreme caution, as dendritic reticulum cells, normal components of the lymph node, express S100 protein. The addition of the more specific anti-MART-1 antibodies is often helpful in these cases.

MART-1 (Melanoma Antigen Recognized by T Cells)
Introduction

MART-1 (melanoma antigen recognized by T cells) is a transmembrane protein that is expressed on melanosomes and is recognized by a subgroup of HLA-A2+ cytotoxic T cells *(10–12)*. It is expressed by normal and malignant melanocytes and cells within the human retina *(13)*. MART-1 elicits a cytotoxic response that has been exploited in the development of immunotherapy protocols for patients with metastatic melanoma. Specifically targeted therapy for patients expressing high levels of MART-1 on their tumor cells is proving to be an effective treatment modality *(14)*. Despite its name, MART-1 has not proven to be specific for melanoma cells, and the same antigen can be detected on benign melanocytes, as well. Very similar antibodies reacting to a slightly different clone, A103 or Melan-A, display similar but not identical staining patterns and will not be discussed further *(15)*.

Diagnostic Utility

Anti-MART-1 is a widely available, commercially prepared antibody that is part of the routine antibody panel in many laboratories. It is very sensitive and relatively specific for identifying melanocytes; however, similar to other melanocyte markers, it does not reliably distinguish benign nevus cells from melanoma cells. Anti-MART-1 has a staining profile that is similar to HMB-45 (Tables 2 and 3). It has been shown to stain essentially all benign nevi and Spitz's nevi and the majority of primary cutaneous mela-

Table 2
Anti- MART-1 Antibody Essentials*

Melanocytic proliferations	Sensitivity
Primary cutaneous melanoma	80–100%
Metastatic melanoma	70–90%
Benign nevi	20–100%
Spitz's nevi	>90%
Dysplastic nevi	<90%
Desmoplastic melanoma	<60%

Other known positively staining tumors

Angiomyolipomas
Lymphangiomyomatosis
Clear cell "sugar" tumors
Sertoli-Leydig tumors of the ovary
Leydig cell tumors of the testis
Adrenocortical carcinomas

*Paraffin-embedded, formalin-fixed tissue, enhanced with microwave heat-induced epitope retrieval .

Table 3
HMB-45 Essentials*

Sensitivity in melanocytic proliferations	
Primary cutaneous melanoma	67–99%
Desmoplastic melanoma	0–16%
Acquired nevi	
Junctional component	100%
Dermal component	Rare
Dysplastic nevi	
Junctional component	100%
Dermal component	>80%
Spitz nevi	100%
Cellular blue nevi	100%
Metastatic melanoma	58–85%

*Formalin-fixed, paraffin-embedded tissue, no pretreatment necessary, cytoplasmic staining.

nomas (Fig. 4) *(16)*. The majority of benign melanocytes express MART-1 whereas the staining is more heterogeneous in melanoma cells *(17)*. Other authors have found MART-1 to be expressed in only a minority of benign melanocytic nevi, especially congenital ones *(18)*.

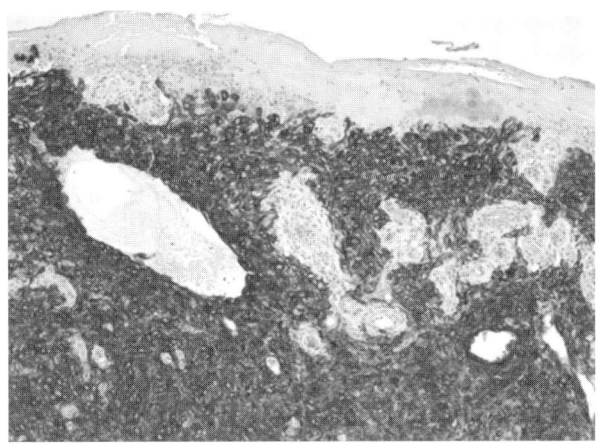

Fig. 4. MART-1 labels virtually all primary cutaneous melanomas.

Sensitivity rates for anti-MART-1 antibodies in detecting primary cutaneous melanomas range from 80 to 100% *(17,18)*. Staining is less reliable for desmoplastic melanomas with sensitivity rates of 60% or lower *(18,19)*. Primary melanomas of the oral mucosa expressed MART-1 in 85% of cases compared with 97% for S100, 94% for tyrosinase, 74% with antimicrophthalmia-associated transcription factor and 71% with HMB-45 *(19)*. In this same study, sinonasal melanomas expressed MART-1 in 100% of cases. Overall, MART-1 expression has been reported to be a less sensitive marker than S100, and similar to HMB-45 and tyrosinase *(20)*.

Metastatic melanoma cells less frequently express MART-1 than do primary cutaneous melanoma cells. However, anti-MART-1 antibodies are more sensitive markers in this situation than is HMB-45, but perhaps less so than anti-tyrosinase antibodies *(16,21)*. Anti-MART-1 antibody stains a higher percentage of cells and with greater intensity than does HMB-45. Sensitivity rates are reported as being from 70–90% for metastatic lesions *(21,22)*. Anti - S100 is the most sensitive marker for detecting metastatic melanoma cells, but is also the least specific of the widely used, commercially available antibodies. Polymerase chain reaction with MART-1 has been used effectively to detect the presence of circulating melanoma cells in patients with localized disease and may convey some prognostic significance *(23,24)*.

MART-1 expression is not limited to melanocytes. It has been demonstrated in angiomyolipomas, lymphangiomyomatosis, clear cell "sugar" tumors and renal capsulomas *(13,25,26)*. Cells in adreno-

cortical neoplasms also express MART-1 and other steroid produc-
ing tumors including Sertoli-Leydig cells tumors of the over and
Leydig cell tumors of the testis *(27)*.

Technical Considerations

Anti-MART-1 antibodies work extremely well on paraffin-
embedded, formalin fixed tissue specimens, as well as on fresh, frozen tissue specimens. They also work well in cytospin specimens
prepared from fine-needle aspirations. Heat-induced epitope retrieval
has shown to improve sensitivity to the levels attained with formalin-
fixed, paraffin-embedded tissue *(12)*. Normal intraepidermal melanocytes serve as a positive internal control for evaluating the
adequacy of the staining procedure.

Summary

Anti-MART-1 is a very useful antibody for the establishing a diagnosis of metastatic melanoma. It is of only limited value for
primary cutaneous melanoma as it does not adequately discriminate
between melanomas and benign melanocytic proliferations. Further,
it is not particularly sensitive for the detection of desmoplastic melanoma. For these reasons, antibodies directed against S100 protein are
probably more useful for establishing neoplastic cells as melanocytic
in primary cutaneous tumors. When looking for metastatic melanoma cells in lymph nodes, anti-MART-1 proves to be much more
specific, though less sensitive than anti-S100, in detecting tumor
cells. A panel including antibodies directed against S100 protein and
MART-1 is useful in maximizing specificity and sensitivity when
trying to establish or detect melanocytic lineage.

HMB-45

Introduction

HMB-45 was introduced in 1986 by Gown et al *(28)*. This antibody
was subsequently found to be localized to the gp100 protein found in
melanosomes within melanoma cells and melanocytes within many
types of benign and atypical nevi *(29)*. The epitope recognized by
HMB-45 is known to be composed, at least in part, of sialic acid *(30)*.
The protein appears to be both inducible and reversible *(31)*. While
originally touted as a "melanoma-specific" antibody, the commercially available products were found to label some benign melanocytes equally well.

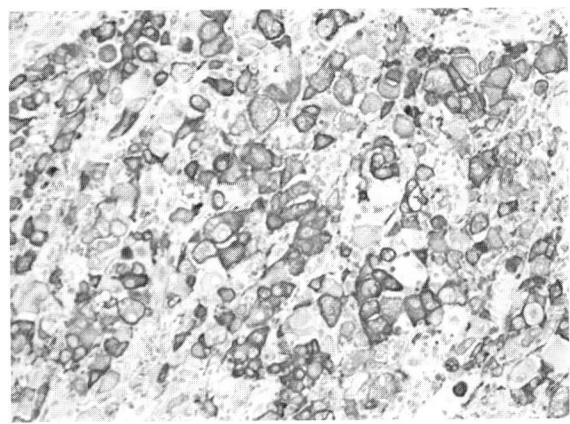

Fig. 5. Most tumor cells in primary cutaneous melanomas express HMB-45.

Diagnostic Utility

Early reports documented HMB-45 labeling of widely disparate neoplasms, including lymphoma, and adenocarcinoma *(32,33)*. It was later suggested that this staining was probably spurious and due to contaminants in the ascites fluid used to produce the first batches of the commercial product *(34)*.

HMB-45 detects melanoma cells within the epidermis and dermis in approximately 92–99% of primary cutaneous melanomas (Fig. 5) *(35–38)*. The staining pattern has been described as strong, but patchy. However, it usually will not recognize the cells in desmoplastic melanomas *(36,39)*. HMB-45 is not specific for melanomas. It has been shown to label melanocytes within dysplastic nevi *(40)*, melanocytes within the epidermis of common nevi and normal melanocytes within fetal skin *(28)*. In addition, HMB-45 labeling is present on melanocytes overlying scars, preventing its use in evaluating adequacy of resection margins *(41)*. Melanocytes within the dermal component of most acquired nevi fail to label with HMB-45; however, dermal melanocytes in Spitz's nevi *(42)*, cellular blue nevi and dysplastic nevi may express the protein recognized by HMB-45 (Table 3) *(36)*.

Approximately 58–85% of metastatic melanomas will be detected by HMB-45 antibody *(37,39,43)*. This is a significantly lower sensitivity rate than other markers such as anti-MART-1, and anti-tyrosinase.

HMB-45 labels only rare nonmelanocytic tumors. It has been consistently demonstrated in angiomylipomas. Rare malignant gastrointestinal stromal tumors have demonstrated HMB-45 positivity

(44). Extensive series generally find few nonmelanocytic tumors expressing the gp100 protein recognized by HMB-45 *(37)*.

Technical Considerations

HMB-45 works well on paraffin-embedded, formalin-fixed tissue. It stains with a diffuse, granular cytoplasmic pattern. The staining pattern is strong, but patchy, with staining intensity often correlated with degree of pigmentation. It is often helpful to use a chromagen other than the brown-staining diaminobenzidine in order to distinguish inherent melanin pigment from true immunolabeling. Normal intraepidermal melanocytes often are labeled by HMB-45 and can serve as an internal positive control to evaluate adequacy of the test. Pretreatment with HIER or enzymatic digestion is not ordinarily required to attain good performance with this antibody.

Summary

HMB-45 antibodies play little role in the diagnosis of a primary cutaneous neoplasm. They are not useful for distinguishing benign from melanocytic proliferations. Anti-S100 protein antibodies are more sensitive and thus, a better choice for determining the melanocytic origin of such a tumor, should this be necessary.

HMB-45 antibodies can serve a useful role as adjunct stains in attempting to identify precisely a metastatic neoplasm. As this marker is more specific than anti-S100 protein, it helps to narrow the differential diagnosis of S100 positive neoplasms. However, it has recently been shown to be somewhat less sensitive than newer markers such as tyrosinase and MART-1 for this purpose, limiting its usefulness *(43,45)*.

Miscellaneous Other Markers

Summary

There are several other commercially available antibodies that can be used for the identification of melanocytic neoplasms. Anti-tyrosinase recognizes the enzyme in melanocytes and has a staining profile similar to that described for MART-1 (Fig. 6) *(43)*. NKI/C3 and anti-microphthalmia transcription factor antibodies similarly appear to offer no specific advantages. NKI/C3 has been shown to react with most atypical fibroxanthomas and dermatofibrosarcoma protuberans, the majority of mesotheliomas, angiomyolipomas, cel-

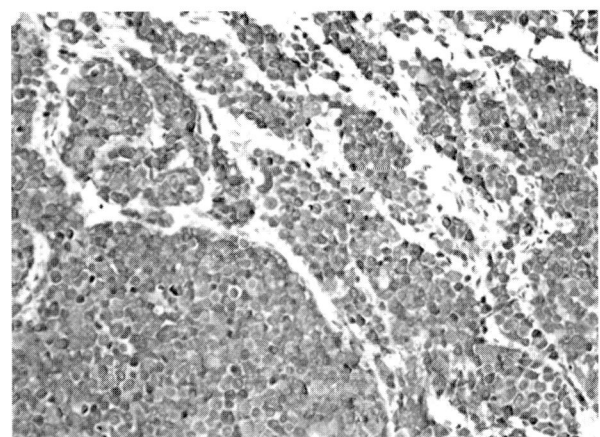

Fig. 6. There is strong cytoplasmic staining of melanocytes within this melanoma stained with anti-tyrosinase antibodies.

lular neurothekeomas, and gastric autonomic nerve tumors *(46–50)*. Microphthalma transcription factor is probably more specific for melanocytic proliferations, but is no more sensitive than the melanoma markers described above. These newer markers appear to offer no definitive advantages in sensitivity or specificity over those described above *(38,39)*. It should be noted, however, that every laboratory attains slightly different results and has varying degrees of success with each antibody. Thus, it is important to select those that perform the most reliably and reproducibly in any given setting.

Newer markers such as anti-MAGE antibodies are purported to be useful in detecting invasive melanomas, but not to label benign melanocytic proliferations or *in situ* melanomas *(51)*. However, there is not yet sufficient data to evaluate the utility of these reagents. SMS-5 antibody is alleged to be very highly sensitive and specific for melanocytic neoplasms, making it a useful marker for precisely identifying metastatic lesions *(37)*, but again, the available data is limited at this time.

References

1. Moore, W. B. (1965) A soluble protein characteristic of the nervous system. *Biochem. Biophys. Res. Commun.* **19,** 739–744.
2. Haimoto, H., Hosada, S., and Kato, K. (1987) Differential distribution of immunoreactive S100-alpha and S100-beta proteins in normal nonnervous human tissues. *Lab. Invest.* **57,** 489–498.

3. McNutt, N. S. (1998) The S100 family of multipurpose calcium-binding proteins. *J. Cutan. Pathol.* **25,** 521–529.
4. Cochran, A. J., Duan-Ren, W., Herschman, H. R., and Gaynor, R. B. (1982) Detection of S-100 protein as an aid to the identification of melanocytic tumors. *Int. J. Cancer* **30,** 295–297.
5. Ordonez, N. G., Xiaolong, J., and Hickey, R. C. (1988) Comparison of HMB-45 monoclonal antibody and S-100 protein in the immunohistochemical diagnosis of melanoma. *Am. J. Clin. Pathol.* **90,** 385–390.
6. Walsh, N. M. G., Roberts, J. T., Orr, W., and Simon, G. T. (1988) Desmoplastic malignant melanoma. *Arch. Pathol. Lab. Med.* **112,** 922–927.
7. Franquemont, D. W. and Mills, S. E. (1991) Sinonasal malignant melanoma. *Am. J. Clin. Pathol.* **96,** 689–697.
8. Argenyi, Z. B., Cain, C., Bromley, C., Van Nguyen, A., Abraham, A. A., Kerschmann, R., and LeBoit, P. E. (1994) S-100 protein-negative malignant melanoma: fact or fiction? A light-microscopic and immunohistochemical study. *Am. J. Dermatopathol.* **16,** 233–240.
9. Gown, A. M., de Wever, N., and Battifora, H. (1993) Microwave-based antigenic unmasking. A revolutionary new technique for routine immunohistochemistry. *Appl. Immunohistochem.* **1,** 256–266.
10. Rivoltini, L., Kawakami, Y., Sakaguchi, K., Southwood, S., Sette, A., Robbins, P. F., et al. (1995) Induction of tumor-reactive CTL from peripheral blood and tumor-infiltrating lymphocytes of melanoma patients by in vitro stimulation with an immunodominant peptide of the human melanoma antigen MART-1. *J. Immunol.* **154,** 2257–2265.
11. Kawakami, Y., Robbins, P. F., and Rosenberg, S. A. (1996) Human melanoma antigens recognized by T lymphocytes. *Keio J. Med.* **45,** 100–108.
12. Fetsch, P. A., Cormier, J., and Hijazi, Y. M. (1997) Immunocytochemical detection o MART-1 in fresh and paraffin-embedded malignant melanomas. *J. Immunother.* **20,** 60–64.
13. Fetsch, P. A., Fetsch, J. F., Marincola, F. M., Travis, W., Batts, K. P., and Abati, A. (1998) Comparison of melanoma antigen recognized by T cells (MART-1) to HMB-45: additional evidence to support a common lineage for angiomyolipoma, lymphangiomyomatosis, and clear cell sugar tumor. *Mod. Pathol.* **11,** 699–703.
14. Reed, J. A. and Albino, A. P. (2000) Update of diagnostic and prognostic markers in cutaneous malignant melanoma. *Clin. Lab. Med.* **20,** 817–838.
15. Shidham, V. B., Qi, D. Y., Acker, S., Kampalath, B., Chang, C. C., George, V., and Komorowski, R. (2001) Evaluation of micrometastases in sentinel lymph nodes of cutaneous melanoma: higher diagnostic accuracy with Melan-A and MART-1 compared with S100 protein and HMB-45. *Am. J. Surg. Pathol.* **25,** 1039–1046.
16. Kageshita, T., Kawakami, Y., Hirai, S., and Ono, T. (1997) Differential expression of MART-1 in primary and metastatic melanoma lesions. *J. Immunother.* **20,** 460–465.
17. Bergman, R., Azzam, H., Sprecher, E., Manov, L., Munichor, M., Friedman-Birnbaum, R., and Ben-Itzhak, O. (2000) A comparative immunohistochemical study of MART-1 expression in Spitz nevi, ordinary melanocytic nevi, and malignant melanomas. *J. Am. Acad. Dermatol.* **42,** 496–500.
18. Mehregan, D. R. and Hamzavi, I. (2000) Staining of melanocytic neoplasms by melanoma antigen recognized by T cells. *Am. J. Dermatopathol.* **22,** 247–250.

19. Prasad, M. L., Jungbluth, A. A., Iversen, K., Huvos, A. G., and Busan, K. J. (2001) Expression of melanocytic differentiation markers in malignant melanoma of the oral and sinonasal mucosa. *Am. J. Surg. Pathol.* **25,** 782–787.

20. de Vries, T. J., Smeets, M., de Graaf, R., Hou-Jensen, K., Brocker, E. B., Renard, N., et al. (2001) Expression of gp100, MART-1, tyrosinase, and S100 in paraffin-embedded primary melanomas and locoregional, lymph node, and visceral metastases: implications for diagonsis and immunotherapy. A study conducted by the EORTC Melanoma Cooperative Group. *J. Pathol.* **193,** 13–20.

21. Cormier, J. N., Abati, A., Fetsch, P. A., Hijazi, Y. M., Rosenberg, S. A., Marincola, F. M., and Topalian, S. L. (1998) Comparative analysis of the in vivo expression of tyrosinase, MART-1/Melan-A, an gp100 in metastatic melanoma lesions: implications for immunotherapy. *J. Immunother.* **21,** 27–31.

22. Fetsch, P. A., Marincola, F. M., Filie, A., Hijazi, Y. M., Kleiner, D. E., and Abati, A. (1999) Melanoma-associated antigen recognized by T cells (MART-1): the advent of a preferred immunocytochemical antibody for the diagnosis of metastatic malignant melnaoma with fine-needle aspiration. *Cancer* **87,** 37–42.

23. Curry, B. J., Myers, K., and Hersey, P. (1999) MART-1 is expressed less frequently on circulating melanoma cells in patients who develop distant compared with locoregional metastases. *J. Clin. Oncol.* **17,** 2562–2571.

24. Curry, B. J., Myers, K., and Hersey, P. (2001) Utility of tests for circulating melanoma cells in identifying patients who develop recurrent melanoma. *Recent Results Cancer Res.* **158,** 211–230.

25. Bonetti, F., Martignoni, G., Colato, C., Manfrin, E., Gambacorta, M., Faleri, M., et al. (2001) Abdominopelvic sarcoma of perivascular epithelioid cells. Report of four cases in young women, one with tuberous sclerosis. *Mod. Pathol.* **14,** 563–568.

26. Jungbluth, A. A., Iversen, K., Coplan, K. A., Williamson, B., Chen, Y. T., Stockert, E., et al. (1999) Expression of melanocyte-associated markers gp-100 and Melan-A/MART-1 in angiomyolipomas. An immunohistochemical and rt-PCR analysis. *Virchows Arch.* **434,** 429–435.

27. Busam, K. J., Iverson, K., Coplan, K. A., Old, L. J., Stockert, E., Chen, Y. T., McGregor, D., and Jungbluth, A. A. (1998) Immunoreactivity for A103, an antibody to melan-A (MART-1), in adrenocortical and other steroid tumors. *Am. J. Surg. Pathol.* **22,** 57–63.

28. Gown, A. M., Vogel, A. M., Hoak, D.H., Gough, F., and McNutt, M.A. (1986) Monoclonal antibodies specific for melanocytic tumors distinguish subpopulatins of melanocytes. *Am. J. Pathol.* **123,** 195–203.

29. Taatjes, D. J., Arendash-Durand, B., von Turkovich, M., and Trainer, T. D. (1993) HMB-45 antibody demonstrates melanosome specificity by immuno-electron microscopy. *Arch. Pathol. Lab. Med.* **117,** 264–268.

30. Kappur, R. P., Bigler, S. J., McGrath, E., Skelly, M., and Gown, A. M. (1991) Anti-melanoma antibody HMB-45 identifies and oncofetal premelanosome-associated glycoprotein. *Lab. Invest.* **64,** 105 (abstract).

31. Smoller, B. R., Hsu, A., and Krueger, J. (1991) HMB-45 monoclonal antibody recognizes an inducible and reversible melanocyte cytoplasmic protein. *J. Cutan. Pathol.* **18,** 315–322.

32. Friedman, H. D. and Tatum, A. H. (1991) HMB-45 positive malignant lymphoma: a case report with literature review of aberrant HMB-45 reactivity. *Arch. Pathol. Lab. Med.* **115,** 826–830.

33. Hancock, C., Allen, B. C., and Herrera, G. A. (1991) HMB-45 detection in adenocarcinomas. *Arch. Pathol. Lab. Med.* **115,** 886–890.
34. Bonetti, F., Pea, M., Martignoni, G., Riva, M., Columbari, R., Mombello, A., et al. (1991) False-positive immunostaining of normal epithelia and carcinomas with ascites fluid preparations of antimelanoma melanoma antiody HMB-45. *Am. J. Clin. Pathol.* **95,** 454–459.
35. Wick, M. R., Swanson, P. E., and Rozamora, A. (1988) Recognition of malignant melanoma by monoclonal antibody HMB-45: an immunohistochemical study of 200 paraffin-embedded cutaneous tumors. *J. Cutan. Pathol.* **15,** 201–207.
36. Skelton, H. G., III, Smith, K. J., Barrett, T. L., Lupton, G. P., and Graham, J. H. (1991) HMB-45 staining in benign and malignant melanocytic lesions. A reflection of cellular activation. *Am. J. Dermatopathol.* **13,** 543–550.
37. Trefzer, U., Rietz, N., Chen, Y. T., Audring, H., Herberth, G., Siegel, P., et al. (2000) SM5-1: a new monoclonal antibody which is highly sensitive and specific for melanocytic lesions. *Arch. Dermatol. Res.* **292,** 583–589.
38. Fernando, S. S., Johnson, S., and Bate, J. (1994) Immunohistochemical analysis of cutaneous malignant melanoma: comparison of S-100 protein, HMB-45 monoclonal antibody and NKI/C3 monoclonal antibody. *Pathology* **26,** 16–19.
39. Orchard, G. E. (2000) Comparison of immunohistochemical labelling of melanocyte differentiation antibodies melan-A, tyrosinase and HMB-45 with NKIC3 and S100 protein in the evaluation of benign naevi and malignant melanoma. *Histochem.* **32,** 475–481.
40. Smoller, B. R., McNutt, N. S., and Hsu, A. (1989) HMB-45 staining of dysplastic nevi. Support for a spectrum of progression toward melanoma. *Am. J. Surg. Pathol.* **13,** 680–684.
41. Smoller, B. R., McNutt, N. S., and Hsu, A. (1988) HMB-45 recognizes stimulated melanocytes. *J. Cutan. Pathol.* **16,** 49–53.
42. Palazzo, J. P. and Duray, P. H. (1988) Congenital agminated Spitz nevi: immunoreactivity with a melanoma associated monoclonal antibody. *J. Cutan. Pathol.* **15,** 166–170.
43. Kaufman, O., Koch, S., Burghardt, J., Audring, H., and Dietel, M. (1998) Tyrosinase, melan-A, and KBA62 as markers for the immunohistochemical identification of metastatic amelanotic melanomas on paraffin sections. *Mod. Pathol.* **11,** 740–746.
44. Orosz, Z. (1999) Melan-/Mart-1 expression in various melanocytic lesions and in nonmelanocytic soft tissue tumours. *Histopathology* **34,** 517–525.
45. Blessing, K., Sanders, D. S., and Grant, J. J. (1998) Comparison of immunohistochemical staining of the novel antibody melan-A with S100 protein and HMB-45 in malignant melanomas and melanoma variants. *Histopathology* **32,** 139–146.
46. Ma, C. K., Zarbo, R. J., and Gown, A. M. (1992) Immunohistochemical characterization of atypical fibroxanthoma and dermatofibrosarcoma protuberans. *Am. J. Clin. Pathol.* **97,** 478–483.
47. Shanks, J. H., Harris, M., Banerjee, S. S., and Eyden, B. P. (1996) Gastrointestinal autonomic nerve tumours: a report of nine cases. *Histopathology* **29,** 111–121.
48. Shanks, J. H., Harris, M., Banerjee, S. S., Eyden, B. P., Joglekar, V. M., Nicol, A., et al. (2000) Mesotheliomas with deciduoid morphology: a morphologic spectrum and a variant not confined to young females. *Am. J. Surg. Pathol.* **24,** 285–294.

49. Stone, C. H., Lee, M. S., Amin, M. B., Yaziji, H., Gown, A. M., Ro, J. Y., et al. (2001) Renal angiomyolipoma: further immunophenotypic characterization of an expanding morphologic spectrum. *Arch. Pathol. Lab. Med.* **125,** 751–758.

50. Chatelain, D., Ricard, J., Colombat, M., Ghighi, C., Thelu, F., Cordonnier, C., et al. (2000) Cellular neurothekeoma, a rare cutaneous tumor. Anatomoclinical and immunohistochemical study of 2 cases. *Ann. Pathol.* **20,** 225–227.

51. Busam, K. J., Iversen, K., Berwick, M., Spagnoli, G. C., Old, L. J., and Jungbluth, A. A. (2000) Immunoreactivity with the anti-MAGE antibody 57B in malignant melanoma: frequency of expression and correlation with prognostic parameters. *Mod. Pathol.* **13,** 459–465.

7 Neuroectodermal (Other than Melanocytic) and Neuroendocrine Markers

Cytokeratin 20

Introduction

Antibodies directed specifically against cytokeratin 20 (CK20) were first reported in 1992 *(1)*. Cytokeratin 20 is a low molecular weight keratin, an intermediate filament restricted to gastrointestinal and urothelial epithelium, and Merkel cells *(2)*. The initial antibodies worked only on frozen tissue specimens and thus had limited diagnostic utility. Subsequent antibodies that recognize epitopes that survive formalin fixation and paraffin embedding have been developed, increasing the functionality of anti-CK20 antibodies as a diagnostic tool.

Diagnostic Utility

While not totally specific for Merkel cell carcinoma, anti-CK20 antibody will label only a limited number of neoplasms within the skin, thus making it an invaluable tool in establishing a diagnosis *(3)*. Anti-CK20 antibodies stain 67–100% of Merkel cell carcinomas *(4–9)*. Two staining patterns are described. The most characteristic pattern is that of a perinuclear, punctate dot of positivity in the cytoplasm, adjacent to the nucleus (Fig. 1). This pattern is seen in up to 90% of Merkel cell carcinomas, but may not be the predominant pattern *(5,10)*. The other staining pattern seen in Merkel cell carcinomas is a membranous pattern at the periphery of tumor cells (Fig. 2). In most Merkel cell carcinomas, the vast majority of cells will stain intensely with this reagent. It has been suggested that CK20 is least likely to be expressed by cells within Merkel cell carcinomas that express chromogranin and/or synaptophysin *(11)*.

Early reports suggested that anti-CK20 antibody staining was exceptional in small cell carcinomas of the lung *(5)*. These authors

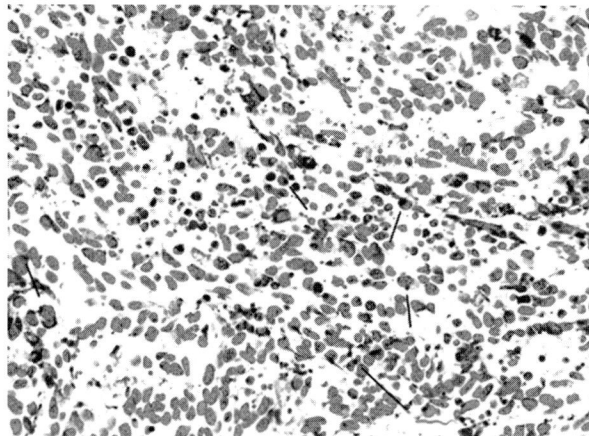

Fig. 1. Punctate, peri-nuclear staining characterizes anti-CK20 in Merkel cell carcinomas. Arrows indicate peri-nuclear dots in some of the tumor cells.

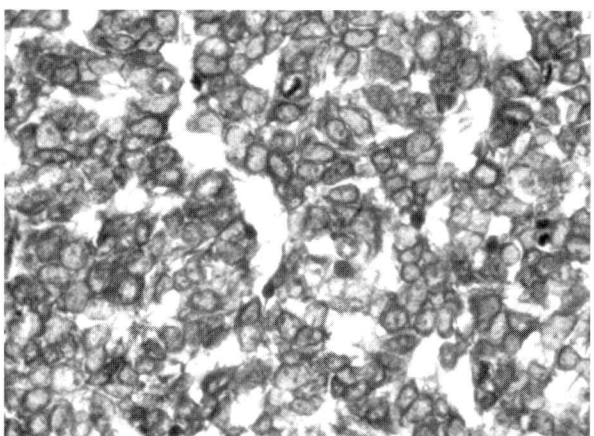

Fig. 2. CK20 may also demonstrate a membranous staining pattern in Merkel cell carcinomas.

believed that staining with anti-CK20 antibodies would serve as a reliable way to distinguish primary cutaneous neuroendocrine carcinomas (Merkel cell carcinomas) from neuroendocrine carcinomas of the lung metastatic to the skin *(5)*. However, subsequent studies have demonstrated strong and diffuse staining of small cell lung carcinomas in up to 33% of cases, thus somewhat tempering the enthusiasm of this antibody for this purpose *(12)*.

Table 1
Essentials of Anti-Cytokeratin 20 Antibodies*

	Sensitivity
Merkel cell carcinoma	67–100%
Other tumors known to express cytokeratin 20	
Colonic adenocarcinoma	<100%
(primary and metastatic)	
Renal oncocytoma	80%
Pancreatic adenocarcinoma	62%
Gastric adenocarcinoma	50%
Cholangiocarcinoma	43%
Small cell carcinoma of the lung	33%
Transitional cell carcinoma of the bladder	29%
Renal cell carcinoma	7%
Hepatocellular carcinoma (focal)	Rare
Mucinous ovarian carcinoma	
Carcinoid (focal)	
Endometrial carcinoma	

*Paraffin-embedded, formalin-fixed tissue. Punctate, perinuclear cytoplasmic staining or membranous staining for Merkel cell carcinoma. Pressure cooking antigen retrieval enhances sensitivity.

Anti-CK20 labels other carcinomas, as is seen in Table 1. However, rarely do these neoplasms enter into the differential diagnosis of a Merkel cell carcinoma based upon routine morphologic features and the clinical presentations *(13)*. One neoplasm that can occasionally present in the skin and cause difficulty in attempting to distinguish it from Merkel cell carcinoma is a primitive neuroectodermal tumor (PNET). PNETs are uniformly negative with anti-CK20 antibodies and almost always express CD99 (*see* CD99 [MIC2] section) *(7)*. Merkel cell carcinomas may also occasionally express CD99, but most often do not *(7)*.

Technical Considerations

Anti-CK20 antibodies work well in formalin-fixed, paraffin-embedded tissue sections. Pretreating the tissue sections with antigen retrieval techniques such as pressure-cooking enhances their sensitivity *(5)*. In our laboratory, we incubate with proteinase K prior to initiating the immunolabeling procedure.

Summary

Anti-CK20 antibodies have a limited, but definite role in diagnostic dermatopathology. Anti-CK20 antibodies have become the first choice antibodies for confirming a diagnosis of Merkel cell carcinoma. The antibody is very sensitive and relatively specific. Its high sensitivity and specifity make this antibody superior to chromogranin and synaptophysin for establishing the diagnosis. When used in conjunction with anti-thyroid transcription factor-1 (which does not label Merkel cell carcinoma), one can now reliably distinguish the primary cutaneous neuroendocrine carcinoma (Merkel cell carcinoma) from small cell carcinoma of the lung metastatic to the skin in most cases (*see* Chapter 9) *(4,8,12)*.

Neuron-Specific Enolase (NSE)

Introduction

An antibody directed against neuron-specific enolase (NSE) was one of the earliest immunomarkers widely used in diagnostic laboratories *(14)*. NSE is an enzyme expressed by neuroendocrine cells. It was thought to be a specific marker for neuroendocrine cells *(15)*. Initial studies reported the effectiveness of NSE expression in distinguishing between Merkel cells and other cells within the epidermis. However, with increasing experience, its lack of specificity has become more apparent, markedly diminishing its diagnostic utility.

Diagnostic Utility

Anti-NSE antibody stains close to 100% of Merkel cell carcinomas (*see* Table 2). The cytoplasmic staining varies in intensity between cells. Nuclei are not stained by this antibody *(15)*.

Anti-NSE is not a specific marker for neuroendocrine cells (*see* Table 2). NSE expression is present in some malignant melanomas *(15)* as well as in benign melanocytic proliferations *(16)*. It is also expressed by neuroblastomas, which also may occasionally present in the skin *(17)*. Some neural tumors, such as cellular neurothekeomas, malignant schwannomas, cutaneous meningiomas and palisaded encapsulated neuromas express NSE *(18–21)*. A majority of cases of Langerhans cell histiocytosis and lymphoepithelioma-like carcinomas of the skin are also recognized with anti-NSE antibodies *(22–24)*. NonX histiocytoses do not express NSE *(24)*.

Table 2
Essentials of Anti-Neuron-Specific Enolase Antibodies*

	Sensitivity
Merkel cell carcinoma	<100%
Other tumors known to express NSE	
Malignant schwannoma	100%
Langerhans cell histiocytosis	70–90%
Neurothekeoma (cellular type)	50%
Palisaded encapsulated neuroma	36%
Lymphoepithelioma-like carcinoma	20%
Chondroid syringoma	
Cutaneous meningioma	
Melanoma	
Benign nevus	
Neuroblastoma	

*Paraffin-embedded, formalin-fixed tissue, cytoplasmic staining.

Technical Considerations

Anti-NSE is a polyclonal antibody that works well on formalin-fixed, paraffin-embedded tissue sections. No pretreatment is necessary. However, the antibody tends to stain with a high degree of background staining. Nerves within the dermis can serve as a positive internal control to evaluate the technical adequacy of the test.

Summary

Anti-NSE antibody has limited utility owing to its relatively low specificity, and has been referred to as "nonspecific" enolase. While it works as a marker for Merkel cell carcinomas, it has largely been supplanted in this role by anti-CK20 (*see* Cytokeratin 20 section), which is more specific. We do not currently use this antibody in our laboratory.

Chromagranin A

Introduction

After its initial recognition, chromogranin rapidly became the most widely used marker for endocrine and neuroendocrine tumors, including Merkel cell carcinomas in the skin *(25)*. Chromogranin A is located within the neurosecretory granules of neuroendocrine cells

Table 3

Anti-Chromogranin A Antibody Essentials*

	Sensitivity
Merkel cell carcinomas	30–70%
Other tumors known to express chromogranin A	
Primary mucinous eccrine carcinoma	
Neurothekeoma	Rare
Malignant peripheral nerve sheath tumor	Rare
Metastatic neuroendocrine carcinoma	Common

*Paraffin-embedded, formalin-fixed tissue, granular, cytoplasmic staining pattern, patchy staining in tumors.

(26). Individual Merkel cells normally found within the epidermis express chromogranin A. Chromogranin B was not found in Merkel cell carcinomas *(25).*

Diagnostic Utility

Anti-chromogranin A antibodies label Merkel cell carcinomas and other neuroendocrine tumors with a granular cytoplasmic pattern, identifying the protein within neurosecretory granules *(27).* However, chromogranin A is found in only a small percentage of tumor cells in positive cases *(28).* In addition, the protein is not detected in many cases, with the reported sensitivity rates ranging from 30–70% *(29–31).*

Chromogranin A is expressed by other neural tumors in the skin, none of which would be in the histologic differential diagnosis of Merkel cell carcinoma (Table 3). These tumors include primary mucinous eccrine carcinomas, a minority of cellular neurothekeomas, and occasional malignant peripheral nerve sheath tumors *(32–34).* In all cases, however, there are antibodies that are more useful in arriving at these diagnoses than anti-chromogranin A. While not totally specific for Merkel cell carcinomas, the presence of chromogranin A positivity in a primary cutaneous neoplasm with histologic features of a Merkel cell carcinoma would certainly be strong confirmatory evidence. However, neuroendocrine carcinomas metastatic to the skin would not be excluded based upon this finding *(35).*

Technical Considerations

Anti-chromogranin A antibodies work well on formalin-fixed, paraffin-embedded tissue sections. The antibody labels appropriate

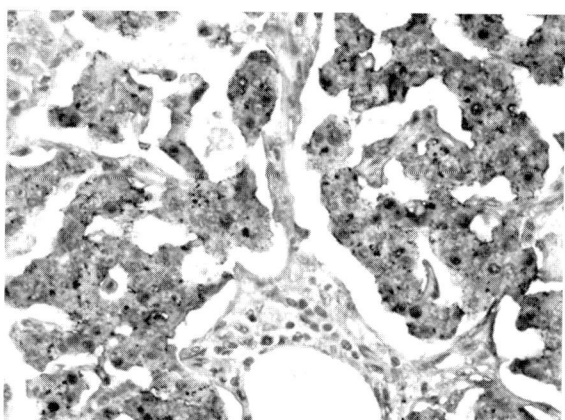

Fig. 3. Anti-chromogranin antibodies often demonstrate a high level of background staining.

cells with a granular, cytoplasmic pattern. The antigen survives routine processing, despite the fact that such processing will often destroy the neurosecretory granules that produce this protein *(30)*. One drawback is that the antibody tends to have a high level of background staining sometimes making interpretation difficult (Fig. 3). HIER has been shown to increase staining intensity *(36)*.

Summary

Anti-chromogranin A antibodies have become less useful in the work-up of a Merkel cell carcinoma with the widespread availability of anti-cytokeratin 20 antibodies. While anti-chromogranin A antibodies are relatively specific for Merkel cell carcinomas (within the differential diagnosis of "blue cell tumors" in the skin), they are far less sensitive than anti-cytokeratin 20 antibodies *(37)*. It has been suggested that the combined use of anti-CK20 and anti-chromogranin antibodies enhances the sensitivity in accurately diagnosing Merkel cell carcinoma *(11)*.

Synaptophysin
Introduction

Synaptophysin is found in presynaptic vesicles and has been detected in neurons, neuroendocrine cells and neoplasms derived from these cell populations *(38)*. It is an integral membrane glycoprotein *(39)*. It is found within dense core granules as well as synaptic vesicles *(40)*.

Table 4
Anti-Synaptophysin Antibody Essentials*

	Sensitivity
Merkel cell carcinoma	29–94%
Other tumors known to express synaptophysin	
Cutaneous primitive neuroectodermal tumor	25%
Malignant peripheral nerve sheath tumor	Rare
Neurofollicular hamartoma	
Neuroblastoma	
Ganglioneuroblastoma	
Ganglioneuroma	
Pheochromocytoma	
Paraganglioma	
Islet cell neoplasms	
Medullary thyroid carcinoma	
Carcinoid	

*Paraffin-embedded, formalin-fixed tissue, cytoplasmic and membranous staining.

Diagnostic Utility

Synaptophysin is detected in up to 29–94% of Merkel cell carcinomas *(29,40)*. However, it is not specific for Merkel cell tumors (Table 4). Other neural and neuroendocrine neoplasms including malignant peripheral nerve sheath tumors, cutaneous peripheral neuroectodermal tumors and neurofollicular hamartomas express this protein *(39, 41–43)*. Synaptophysin expression has not been detected in melanomas *(39)*. It does not stain other cutaneous neoplasms. This makes the antibody relatively specific in the diagnosis of cutaneous neoplasms.

Technical Considerations

Anti-synaptophysin antibodies that survive routine fixation are commercially available. Membranous staining is apparent in cells with presynaptic and/or dense core secretory vesicles *(39)*. In our laboratory, we routinely incubate the tissue sections with proteinase K prior to initiating immunolabeling procedures. HIER also has been shown to increase staining intensity *(36)*.

Summary

Synaptophysin and chromogranin are not necessarily detected in identical cell populations. Each of these functions as a marker for both neural and neuroendocrine cells, but neither is expressed by all cells in a given tumor. Thus, their combined use increases overall sensitivity in arriving at such a diagnosis. However, when diagnosing Merkel cell carcinoma, for example, cytokeratin 20 is a far more sensitive marker, and thus, has largely replaced the use of these markers in establishing these types of diagnoses.

CD57

Introduction

CD57, also known as leu-7, is an epitope that is present on natural killer cells. It is also found on the inner core cells within Pacinian corpuscles and other neural structures *(44)*.

Diagnostic Utility

Anti-CD57 antibody is a useful tool for the identification of two widely disparate types of cutaneous processes. It can be used to identify natural killer cells in hematopoietic infiltrates, though CD56 is more sensitive for this purpose (*see* Chapter 5). It is also a marker for neuronal differentiation and can be used to define this type of differentiation in tumors (Fig. 4), (Table 5). Some histologic variants of neurofibroma express CD57, as do the nerve fibers in epithelial sheath neuromas, nerve sheath myxomas, palisaded encapsulated neuromas and glial cells in heterotopias *(18,19,45–47)*. Only the neural elements in these lesions express this antigen. CD57 expression has been used to differentiate neurofibromas from neurotized nevi that do not express this antigen *(48)*. It can also be used to differentiate palisaded encapsulated neuromas that contain neuronal elements from schwannomas that ordinarily do not contain many.

CD57 is also expressed on the tumor cells in granular dermatofibromas and occasional myofibroblastic dermatofibromas and fibrous histiocytomas *(49–51)*. This raises the question of the etiology of these neoplasms and their relationship to neural differentiation.

Technical Considerations

Anti-CD57 is an antibody that works well in formalin-fixed, paraffin-embedded tissue. It has a strong signal to noise ratio and very little background staining. In normal skin, nerve fibers can be used as an appropriate positive internal control to evaluate the adequacy of the staining procedure. HIER has been shown to increase staining intensity *(36)*.

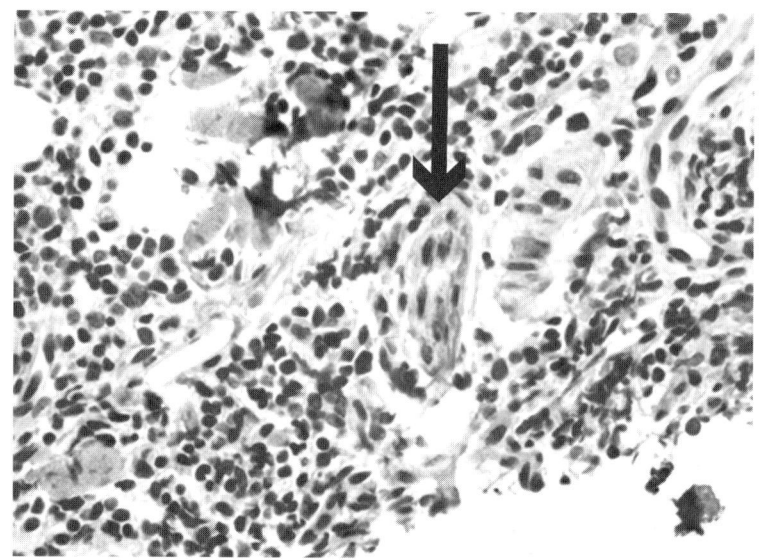

Fig. 4. CD57 is expressed in normal cutaneous nerves. The arrow points to a nerve-expressing CD57.

Table 5
Anti-CD57 Antibody Essentials*

Tumors known to express CD57	Sensitivity
Fibrous histiocytomas	65%
Nerve sheath myxoma (cellular type)	25%
Palisaded encapsulated neuroma	18%
Neurofibroma	Subset
Neuroma	
Myofibroblastic dermatofibroma	
Granular dermatofibroma	

*Paraffin-embedded, formalin-fixed tissue.

Summary

CD57 is a marker with a small, but helpful role in dermatopathology. It is a more specific marker for neuronal elements than is S100 protein, and therefore can be used to identify more precisely neural origin or differentiation in tumors. It is used as a marker for natural killer cells in determining subtypes of lymphoma, though it is less sensitive than CD56 for this purpose (*see* Chapter 5).

Table 6
Use of Immunomarkers in Distinguishing
Benign Cutaneous Neural Neoplasms

	Neurofibroma	Palisaded encapsulated neuroma	Schwannoma	Granular cell tumor
S100 protein	Focally positive	Focally positive	Diffusely positive	Diffusely positive
PGP9.5	Focally positive	Focally positive	Rare positive cells	Positive
CD57	Focally positive	Focally positive	Mostly negative	Mostly negative
Epithelial membrane antigen	Focally positive	Focally positive	Mostly negative	Mostly negative

PGP 9.5

Introduction

PGP 9.5 is a marker for neuroectodermal tissue. The protein is expressed by nerve fibers and in neurons within both the peripheral and central nervous systems.

Diagnostic Utility

Cellular neurothekeomas express PGP 9.5. This is a useful characteristic, as these neoplasms most commonly fail to label with any other antibodies *(11)*. Granular cell tumors express PGP 9.5 in virtually 100% of cases *(52,53)*. Similarly, malignant peripheral nerve sheath tumors uniformly express this protein. All benign neural neoplasms that contain neuronal elements will have some PGP9.5 positive cells, which can be helpful in making a distinction between some histologically similar entities (*see* Table 6).

Unfortunately, anti-PGP 9.5 has a relatively low specificity. PGP 9.5 is expressed by up to 50% of basal cell carcinomas, 60% of trichoepitheliomas, 80% of dermatofibromas, and 100% of some types of eccrine neoplasms *(11)*. Merkel cell carcinomas express PGP 9.5 in up to 88% of cases *(54)*.

Melanomas do not ordinarily express PGP 9.5 *(55)*.

Technical Considerations

There are commercially available antibodies directed against PGP 9.5. These antibodies require no pretreatment and work well on formalin-fixed, paraffin-embedded tissue sections. However, in our laboratory, we have increased the sensitivity of these antibodies with HIER pretreatment.

Summary

At this point, there is little use for anti-PGP 9.5 antibodies in a diagnostic dermatopathology laboratory. The antibodies may be useful in confirming the neuroectodermal nature of a neoplasm, but in most cases, this can be done with other antibodies (i.e., anti-S100, anti-NSE). Anti-PGP 9.5 can be helpful in making a diagnosis of cellular neurothekeoma, but due to lack of specificity, any results should be interpreted with caution.

CD99 (MIC2)

Introduction

Anti-CD99 recognizes the p30/32MIC-2 gene product *(56)*. This protein was originally described in neoplastic cells of acute lymphoblastic leukemia, and has subsequently been detected in a wide range of other cells. It has been shown that CD99 can be negatively regulated by the latent membrane protein-1 of the Epstein-Barr virus and upregulated by Sp1 through the nuclear factor-kappa B *(57)*. It may play a role in caspase-independent death of T lymphocytes *(58)*.

Diagnostic Utility

CD99 was first used in dermatopathology as a marker for primitive neuroectodermal tumors (PNETs) (Fig. 5). However, it was shown subsequently that CD99 also labels a significant minority of Merkel cell tumors, a major tumor in the differential diagnosis of PNETs *(see* Table 7) *(7)*. Nonetheless, in conjunction with CD20 (which labels the vast majority of Merkel cell carcinomas, but not PNETs), it still serves a useful purpose for the evaluation of small blue cell tumors, especially in pediatric patients. Cells within extraskeletal Ewing's sarcoma may also express CD99, and this provides a more challenging differential diagnosis, though many authors regard these tumors as identical to PNETs *(59)*.

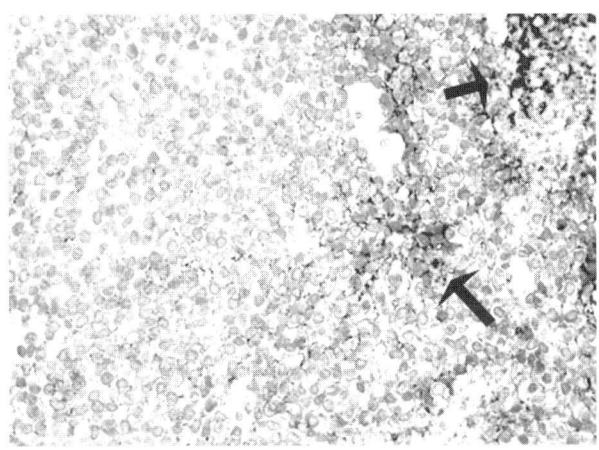

Fig. 5. Primitive neuroectodermal tumors strongly and diffusely express CD99.

Table 7
Anti-CD99 Antibody Essentials*

Tumors known to express CD99	Sensitivity
Primitive neuroectodermal tumor	100%
Acute lymphoblastic leukemia	100%
Acute myelogenous leukemia	80%
Solitary fibrous tumor	75%
Merkel cell carcinoma	40%
Kaposiform hemangioendothelioma	
Juvenile fibromatoses	
Spindle cell epithelioma of the vagina	

*Paraffin-embedded, formalin-fixed tissue.

Cells in acute lymphoblastic lymphoma express CD99. Anti-CD99 antibody labels close to 100% of these neoplasms when they involve the skin (60). However, it also identifies leukemia cells in up to 80% of cases of acute myelogenous leukemia. Thus, CD99 appears to be a sensitive marker for cutaneous leukemia, but does not help in the further subtyping and classification (56). A more elaborate antibody panel is also necessary to distinguish between PNETs and lymphoblastic lymphomas, especially in children (61). A panel with many hematopoietic markers would likely make this distinction in most cases (see Chapter 5).

The scope of tumors identified by CD99 is constantly enlarging and now includes juvenile fibromatoses, solitary fibrous tumors and Kaposiform hemangioendotheliomas (Table 7) *(62–65)*.

Technical Considerations

Antibodies directed against CD99 are very useful on paraffin-embedded, formalin-fixed tissue sections. They will also recognize the epitopes on tissue that has been decalcified, which may be helpful in the work-up of leukemias, as bone marrow biopsies usually require decalcification prior to routine processing and immunolabeling. No pretreatment is necessary when using these antibodies.

Summary

Anti-CD99 antibodies have a very limited role in diagnostic dermatopathology. They can be used in a panel of antibodies to confirm that a small, blue cell tumor represents a primitive neuroectodermal tumor. As these neoplasms are exceedingly rare in the skin, the antibody is not necessarily essential for routine immunopathology in the skin. It is more widely used and necessary in distinguishing between histologically similar neoplasms in a pediatric population.

Other Neuroendocrine Markers

Calcitonin and bombesin are just a couple of the myriad other markers for neuroendocrine cells available in the market. Neither of these immunostains offers any advantages, with lower specificity and/or sensitivity rates than those described above. We do not currently stock any of these additional markers in our laboratory.

References

1. Moll, R., Lowe, A., Laufer, J., and Franke, W. W. (1992) Cytokeratin 20 in human carcinomas. A new histodiagnostic marker detected by monoclonal antibodies. *Am. J. Pathol.* **140,** 427–447.
2. Zemer, R., Fishman, A., Bernheim, J., Zimlichman, S., Markowicz, O., Altaras, M., and Klein, A. (1998) Expression of cytokeratin-20 in endometrial carcinoma. *Gynecol. Oncol.* **70,** 410–413.
3. Miettinen, M. (1995) Keratin 20: immunohistochemical marker for gastrointestinal, urothelial, and Merkel cell carcinomas. *Mod. Pathol.* 8, 384–388.
4. Byrd-Gloster, A. L., Khoor, A., Glass, L. F., Messina, J. L., Whitsett, J. A., Livingston, S. K., and Cagle, P. T. (2000) Differential expression of thyroid transcription factor 1 in small cell lung carcinoma and Merkel cell tumor. *Hum. Pathol.* **31,** 58–62.

5. Chan, J. K., Suster, S., Wenig, B. M., Tsang, W. Y., Chan, J. B., and Lau, A. L. (1997) Cytokeratin immunoreactivity distinguishes Merkel cell (primary cutaneous neuroendocrine) carcinoma and salivary small cell carcinomas from small cell carcinomas of various sites. *Am. J. Surg. Pathol.* **21,** 226–234.

6. Scott, M. P. and Helm, K. F. (1999) Cytokeratin 20: a marker for diagnosis Merkel cell carcinoma. *Am. J. Dermatopathol.* **21,** 16–20.

7. Nicholson, S. A., McDermott, M. B., Swanson, P. E., and Wick, M. R. (2000) CD99 and cytokeratin-20 in small-cell and basaloid tumors of the skin. Appl. Immunohistochem. *Molecul. Morphol.* **8,** 37–41.

8. Cheuk, W., Kwan, M. Y., Suster, S., and Chan, J. K. (2001) Immunostaining for thyroid transcriptin factor 1 and cytokeratin 20 aids the distinction of small cell carcinoma from Merkel cell carcinoma, but not pulmonary from extrapulmonary small cell carcinomas. *Arch. Pathol. Lab. Med.* **125,** 228–231.

9. Stopyra, G. A., Worhol, M. J., and Multhaupt, H. A. (2001) Cytokeratin 20 immunoreactivity in renal oncocytomas. J. Histochem. *Cytochem.* **49,** 19–20.

10. Jensen, K., Kohler, S., and Rouse, R. V. (2000) Cytokeratin staining in Merkel cell carcinoma: an immunohistochemical study of cytokeratins 5/6, 7/17, and 20. *Appl. Immunohistochem. Molecul. Morphol.* **8,** 310–315.

11. Perveen, N., Ma, C. K., Linden, M. D., Zarbo, R. J., and Lee, M. W. (2001) Possible inverse relationsihp of cytokeratin and neuroendocrine markers in Merkel cell carcinoma (abstract). *J. Cutan. Pathol.* **28,** 580.

12. Hanly, A. J., Elgart, G. W., Jorda, M., Smith, J., and Nadji, M. (2000) Analysis of thyroid transcription factor-1 and cytokeratin 20 separates merkel cell carcinoma from small cell carcinoma of the lung. *J. Cutan. Pathol.* **27,** 118–120.

13. Chu, P., Wu, E., and Weiss, L. M. (2000) Cytokeratin 7 and cytokeratin 20 expression in epithelial neoplasms: a survey of 435 cases. *Mod. Pathol.* **13,** 962–972.

14. Gu, J., Polak, J. M., Tapia, F. J., Marangos, P. J., and Pearse, A. G. (1981) Neuron-specific enolase in the Merkel cells of mammalian skin. The use of specific antibody as a simple and reliable histologic marker. *Am. J. Pathol.* **104,** 63–68.

15. Gu, J., Polak, J. M., Van Noorden, S., Pearse, A. G., Marangos, P. J., and Azzopardi, J.G. (1983) Immunostaining of neuron-specific enolase as a diagnostic tool for Merkel cell tumors. *Cancer* **15,** 1039–1043.

16. Dhillon, A. P. and Rode, J. (1982) Patterns of staining for neurone specific enolase in benign and malignant melanocytic lesions of the skin. *Diagn. Histopathol.* **5,** 169–174.

17. Dhillon, A. P., Rode, J., and Leathem, A. (1982) Neurone specific enolase: an aid to the diagnosis of melanoma and neuroblastoma. *Histopathology* **6,** 81–92.

18. Argenyi, Z. B., LeBoit, P. E., Santa Cruz, D., Swanson, P. E., and Kutzner, H. (1993) Nerve sheath myxoma (neurothekeoma) of the skin: light microscopic and immunohistochemical reappraisal of the cellular variant. J. Cutan. Pathol. 20, 294–303.

19. Argenyi, Z. B. (1990) Immunohistochemical characterization of palisaded, encapsulated neuroma. *J. Cutan. Pathol.* **17,** 329–335.

20. Kikuchi, A., Akiyama, M., Han-Yaku, H., Shimizu, H., Naka, W., and HNishikawa, T. (1993) Solitary cutaneous malignant schwannoma. Immunohistochemical and ultrastructural studies. *Am. J. Dermatopathol.* **15,** 15–19.

21. Argenyi, Z. B., Thiberg, M. D., Hayes, C. M., and Whitaker, D. C. 1994, Primary cutaneous meningioma associated with von Recklinghausen's disease. *J. Cutan. Pathol.* **21,** 549–556.

22. Ornvold, K., Nielsen, M. H., and Clausen, N. (1985) Disseminated histiocytosis X. A clinical and immunohistochemical retrospective study. *Acta Pathol. Microbiol. Immunol. Scand. (A)* **93,** 311–316.

23. Swanson, S. A., Cooper, P. H., Mills, S. E., and Wick, M. R. (1988) Lymphoepithelioma-like carcinoma of the skin. *Mod. Pathol.* **1,** 359–365.

24. Kanitakis, J., Fantini, F., Pincelli, C., Hermier, C., Schmitt, D., and Thivolet, J. (1991) Neuron-specific enolase is a marker of cutaneous Langerhans' cell histiocytosis ("X") - a comparative study with S100 protein. *Anticancer Res.* **11,** 635–639.

25. Wiler, R., Fischer-Colbrie, R., Schmid, K. W., Feichtinger, H., Bussolati, G., Grimelius, L., et al. (1988) Immunological studies on the occurrence and properties of chromogranin A and B and secretogranin II in endocrine tumors. *Am. J. Surg. Pathol.* **12,** 877–884.

26. Silver, M. M., Lines, L. D., and Hearn, S. S. (1993) Immunogold detection of chromogranin A in the neuroendocrine tumor. *Ultrastruct. Pathol.* **17,** 83–92.

27. Mount, S. L. and Taatjes, D. J. (1994) Neuroendocrine carcinoma of the skin (Merkel cell carcinoma). An immunoelectron-microscopic case study. *Am. J. Dermatopathol.* **16,** 60–65.

28. Lanzafame, S. (1990) Molecular characterization of cutaneous neuroendocrine (Merkel cell) carcinoma. Review of the literature and presentation of a caseload. *Pathologica* **82,** 257–269.

29. Visscher, D., Cooper, P. H., Zarbo, R. J., and Crissman, J. D. (1989) Cutaneous neuroendocrine (Merkel cell) carcinoma: an immunophenotypic, clinicopathologic, and flow cytometric study. *Mod. Pathol.* **2,** 331–338.

30. Haneke, E., Schulze, H. J., and Marhle, G. (1993) Immunohistochemical and immunoelectron microscopic demonstration of chromogranin A in formalin-fixed tissue of Merkel cell carcinoma. *J. Am. Acad. Dermatol.* **28,** 222–226.

31. Fukunaga, M. and Shinozaki, N. (1995) Immunohistochemical and flow cytometric study of neuroendocrine carcinoma of the skin. *Pathol. Int.* **45,** 513–519.

32. Karabela-Bouropoulou, V., Antoniou, D., and Liapi-Avgeri, G. (1996) Malignant peripheral nerve sheath tumor with glandular differentiation. Report of a case with emphasis to the usefulness of immunohistochemistry in the differential diagnosis. *Arch. Anat. Cytol. Pathol.* **44,** 263–268.

33. Chang, S. E., Lee, T. J., Ro, J. Y., Choi, J. H., Sung, K. J., Moon, K. C., and Koh, J. K. (1999) Cellular neurothekeoma with possible neuroendocrine differentiation. *J. Dermatol.* **26,** 363–367.

34. Bellezza, G., Sidoni, A., and Bucciarelli, E. (2000) Primary mucinous carcinoma of the skin. *Am. J. Dermatopathol.* **22,** 166–170.

35. Yoshimasu, T., Yamamoto, Y., Uede, K., and Furukawa, F. (2001) Skin metastasis of neuroendocrine carcinoma derived form the mediastinum. *J. Dermatol.* **28,** 168–171.

36. Gown, A. M., de Wever, N., and Battifora, H. (1993) Microwave-based antigenic unmasking. A revolutionary new technique for routine immunohistochemistry. *Appl. Immunohistochem.* **1,** 256–266.

37. Moll, I., Kuhn, C., and Moll, R. (1995) Cytokeratin 20 is a general marker of cutaneous Merkel cells while certain neuronal proteins are absent. *J. Invest. Dermatol.* **104,** 910–915.

38. Ortonne, J. P., Petchot-Bacque, J. P., Verrando, P., Pisani, A., Pautrat, G., and Bernerd, F. (1988) Normal Merkel cells express a synaptophysin-like immunoreactivity. *Dermatologica* **177,** 1–10.

39. Gould, V. E., Wiedenmann, B., Lee, I., Schwechheimer, K., Dockhorn-Dworniczak, B., Radosevich, J. A., et al. (1987) Synaptophysin expression in neuroendocrine neoplasms as determined by immunocytochemistry. *Am. J. Pathol.* **126,** 243–257.

40. Buffa, R., Rindi, G., sessa, F., Gini, A., Capella, C., Jahn, R., BNavone, F., De Camilli, P., and Solcia, E. (1987) Synaptophysin immunoreactivity and small clear vesicles in neuroendocrine cells and related tumours. *Mol. Cell. Probes.* **1,** 367–381.

41. Morgan, M. B., Stevens, L., Patterson, J., and Tannenbaum, M. (2000) Cutaneous epithelioid malignant nerve sheath tumor with rhabdoid features: a histologic, immunohistochemical, and ultrastructural study of three cases. *J. Cutan. Pathol.* **27,** 529–534.

42. Xie, D. L., Nielsen, T. A., Pellegrini, A. E., and Hessel, A. B. (1999) Neurofollicular hamartoma with strong diffuse S100 positivity: a case report. *Am. J. Dermatopathol.* **21,** 253–255.

43. Banerjee, S. S., Agbamu, D. A., Eyden, B. P., and Harris, M. (1997) Clinicopathological characteristics of peripheral primitive neuroectodermal tumour of the skin and subcutaneous tissue. *Histopathology* **31,** 355–366.

44. Vega, J. A., Del Valle, M. E., Haro, J. J., Naves, F. J., Calzada, B., and Uribelarrea, R. (1994) The inner-core, outer-core and capsule cells of the human Pacinian corpuscles: an immunohistochemical study. *Eur. J. Morphol.* **32,** 11–18.

45. Michal, M., Fanburg-Smith, J. C., Mentzel, T., Kutzner, H., Requena, L., Zamecnik, M., and Miettinen, M. (2001) Dendritic cell neurofibroma with pseudorosettes: a report of 18 cases of a distinct and hitherto unrecognized neurofibroma variant. *Am. J. Surg. Pathol.* **25,** 587–594.

46. Requena, L., Grosshans, E., Kutzner, H., Ryckaert, C., Cribier, B., Resnik, K. S., and LeBoit, P. E. (2000) Epithelial sheath neuroma: a new entity. *Am. J. Surg. Pathol.* **24,** 190–196.

47. Skelton, H. G., III and Smith, K. J. (1999) Glial heterotopia in the subcutaneous tissue overlying T-12. *J. Cutan. Pathol.* **26,** 523–527.

48. Hwang, S. M., Choi, E. H., Lee, W. S., Choi, S. I., and Ahn, S. K. (1997) Nevus spilus (speckled lentignous nevus) associated with a nodular neurotized nevus. *Am. J. Dermatopathol.* **19,** 308–311.

49. Zelger, B. G., Steiner, H., Kutzner, H., Rutten, A., and Zelger, B. (1997) Granular cell dermatofibroma. *Histopathology* **31,** 258–262.

50. Zelger, B. G., Steiner, H., Kutzner, H., Rutten, A., and Zelger, B. (1997) Verocay body-prominent cutaneous schwannoma. *Am. J. Dermatopathol.* **19,** 242–249.

51. Zelger, B. W., Zelger, B. G., Steiner, H., and Ofner, D. (1996) Aneurysmal and haemangiopericytoma-like fibrous histiocytoma. *J. Clin. Pathol.* **49,** 313–318.

52. Williams, H. K. and Williams, D. B. (1997) Oral granular cell tumours: a histological and immunocytochemical study. *J. Oral Pathol. Med.* **26,** 164–169.

53. Mahalingam, M., LoPiccolo, D., and Byers, H. R. (2001) Expression of PGP 9.5 in granular cell nerve sheath tumors: an immunohistochemical study of six cases. *J. Cutan. Pathol.* **28,** 282–286.

54. Heenan, P. J., Cole, J. M., and Spagnolo, D. V. (1990) Primary cutaneous neuroendocrine carcinoma (Merkel cell carcinoma). An adnexal epithelial neoplasm. *Am. J. Dermatopathol.* **12,** 7–16.

55. Sinkre, P., Yen Moore, A., and Cockerell, C. J. (2001) Expression of PGP 9.5 in desmplastic melanomas: an immunohistochemical study of five cases (abstract). *J. Cutan. Pathol.* **28,** 586.

56. Dorfman, D. M., Kraus, M., Perez-Atayde, A. R., Barnhill, R. L., Pinkus, G. S., and Granter, S. R. (1997) CD99 (p30/32MIC2) immunoreactivity in the diagnosis of leukemia cutis. *Mod. Pathol.* **10,** 283–288.

57. Lee, I., Kim, M. K., Choi, E. Y., Mehl, A., Jung, K. C., Gil, M. C., et al. (2001) CD99 expression is positively regulated by Sp1 and is negatively regulated by Epstein-Barr virus latent membrane protein 1 through nuclear factor-kappaB. *Blood* **97,** 3596–3604.

58. Pettersen, R. D., Bernard, G., Olafsen, M. K., Pourtein, M., and Lie, S. O. (2001) CD99 signals caspase-independent T cell death. *J. Immunol.* **166,** 4931–4942.

59. Boor, A., Jurkovic, I., Friedmann, I., Plank, L., and Kocan, P. (2001) Extraskeletal Ewing's sarcoma of the nose. *J. Laryngol. Otol.* **115,** 74–76.

60. Chimenti, S., Fink-Puches, R., Peris, K., Pescarmona, E., Putz, B., Kerl, H., and Cerroni, L. (1999) Cutaneous involvement in lymphoblastic lymphoma. *J. Cutan. Pathol.* **26,** 379–385.

61. Lucas, D. R., Bentley, G., Dan, M. E., Tabaczka, P., Poulik, J. M., and Mott, M. P. (2001) Ewing sarcoma vs. lymphoblastic lymphoma. A comparative immunohistochemical study. *Am. J. Clin. Pathol.* **115,** 11–17.

62. Fetsch, J. F., Miettinen, M., Laskin, W. B., Michal, M., and Enzinger, F. M. (2000) A clinicopathologic study of 45 pediatric soft tissue tumors with an admixture of adipose tissue and fibroblastic elements, and a proposal for classification as lipofibromatosis. *Am. J. Surg. Pathol.* **24,** 1491–1500.

63. Alawi, F., Stratton, D., and Freedman, P. D. (2001) Solitary fibrous tumor of the oral soft tissues: a clinicopathologic and immunohistochemical study of 16 cases. *Am. J. Surg. Pathol.* **25,** 900–910.

64. Zamecnik, M., Mikleova, Z., and Michal, M. (2000) Kaposiform hemangioendothelioma in adult. Report of a case with amianthoid-like fibrosis and angiectases. *Cesk. Patol.* **36,** 163–167.

65. Skelton, H. G., III and Smith, K. J. (2001) Spindle cell epithelioma of the vagina shows immunohistochemical staining supporting its origin from a primitive/progenitor cell population. *Arch. Pathol. Lab. Med.* **125,** 547–550.

8 Antibodies Used to Identify Infectious Diseases

Herpes Virus

Introduction

There are antibodies directed against herpes virus proteins. Early efforts produced antibodies with extensive cross-reactivity between subtypes of herpes virus and with varicella viruses. In recent years, more specific antibodies directed against specific members of this virus family have been developed.

Diagnostic Utility

Antibodies directed against herpes virus types 1 and 2 could be used in order to increase the sensitivity of making a diagnosis of herpetic dermatitis in cases without blisters or vesicles (Fig. 1A,B). In some cases, antibodies detect the viral antigens, although morphologic changes of herpetic infection of keratinocytes and within nerves cannot be observed *(1,2)*. Tzanck smears and direct immuofluorescence tests performed on cytologic preparations are thought to have a higher sensitivity in establishing a diagnosis of herpes infection than do tissue sections stained with anti-herpes virus antibodies. However, these techniques cannot reliably distinguish between herpes virus types 1 and 2 *(3,4)*. In recent years, specific antibodies directed against herpes virus types 1 and 2 have been developed, permitting distinction between these organisms that cannot be made on routine histologic sections *(4)*. As lesions age, herpes antigen load diminishes, lessening the likelihood of a positive immunostain *(4)*.

Newer antibodies have been developed against specific proteins in the envelope of varicella zoster virus. This protein is not present in herpes simplex virus and thus enables discrimination between herpes infection and varicella infection on paraffin-embedded, formalin-fixed tissue sections *(5)*.

Antibodies directed against human herpes virus 8 (HHV-8) have become commercially available in recent years. HHV-8 has been

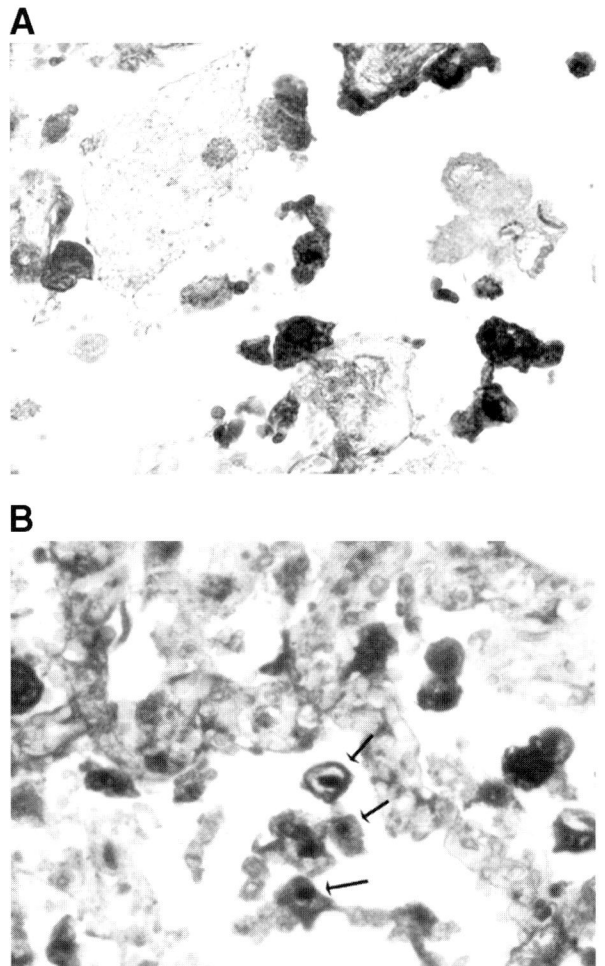

Fig. 1. (A) Anti-herpes antibodies label viral particles in keratinocytes in cases of herpetic dermatitis. Staining can be seen in cases where routine histologic sections may not demonstrate viral inclusions. The positive cells were acantholytic keratinocytes within a blister cavity. **(B)** Intranuclear herpetic inclusions stain very strongly with the antibody. Arrows demonstrate the intranuclear inclusions.

detected in most cases of endemic and epidemic Kaposi's sarcoma *(6)*. In contrast, other cutaneous vascular proliferations are rarely found to contain herpes virus particles *(7,8)*. Some laboratories are using anti-HHV8 staining as a diagnostic tool in distinguishing Kaposi's sarcoma from other spindle vascular proliferations *(9)*.

Anti-herpes virus 6 has been implicated in causing exanthema subitum. Based upon the findings of staining with HHV6 in affected skin, it has also been implicated in the pathogenesis of pityriasis rosea and some cases of erythroderma *(10)*. However, the specificity of these results has been questioned and the antibodies are not routinely used in diagnostic dermatopathology.

Technical Considerations

Antibodies directed against the herpes family viruses are widely available. These antibodies recognize epitopes that survive routine processing and are useful in detecting the present of herpes virus particles in the skin. There is still some concern about extensive cross reactivity, however, and in most cases, it is not yet advisable to attempt to distinguish type 1 from type 2 herpes based upon immunostaining results. Anti-herpes antibodies do not require pretreatment with enzymatic digestion or HIER.

Summary

Anti-herpes virus antibody is a useful tool for identifying the presence of herpes infection on biopsies where no inclusions can be found on routine tissue sections. I do not believe that it is prudent, yet, to rely too heavily on viral subtyping based upon immunostaining profiles.

Cytomegalovirus
Introduction

Cutaneous disease resulting from cytomegalovirus infection (CMV) is quite rare. Thus, there is little need for immunostaining to establish a diagnosis of cutaneous CMV infection in the routine dermatopathology practice. Nonetheless, antibodies directed against different portions of the viral proteins have been developed. Antibodies against early and late antigens are available commercially *(11)*.

Diagnostic Utility

Anti-CMV antibodies can be used to detect CMV organisms in the skin. This is helpful in cases with morphologic features suspicious for CMV, especially in immunosuppressed patients in whom the presence of such organisms may give rise to clinical disease (Fig. 2) *(2)*. CMV inclusions are seen with immunostaining in endothelial cells and fibroblasts, as would be expected *(12)*.

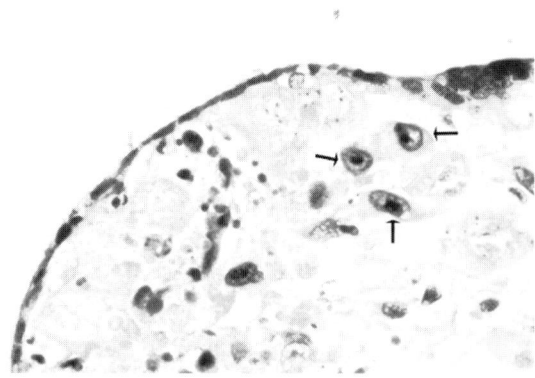

Fig. 2. CMV particles may be found in endothelial cells, especially in immunosuppressed patients. In this placenta, strong nuclear and cytoplasmic staining is seen within stromal cells. Arrows point to intranuclear inclusions that stain strongly positive with this antibody.

Technical Considerations

Antibodies that are directed against early and late CMV antigens are commercially available. These antibodies recognize proteins that survive routine processing *(11)*. Pretreating tissue sections with proteinase K enhances the performance of these antibodies.

Summary

While the technology to identify CMV in routinely fixed skin biopsies is available, there is generally very little clinical need for this test. Therefore, except in laboratories that see large numbers of biopsies from immunosuppressed patients, there is probably little need to have this antibody as part of the general stock.

Epstein-Barr Virus

Introduction

There are antibodies directed against various portions of the Epstein-Barr virus (EBV). The most commonly used one is directed against the latent membrane protein-1 (LMP-1).

Diagnostic Utility

Direct cutaneous infection with EBV does not result in any recognized specific dermatosis. EBV is known to play a role in the patho-

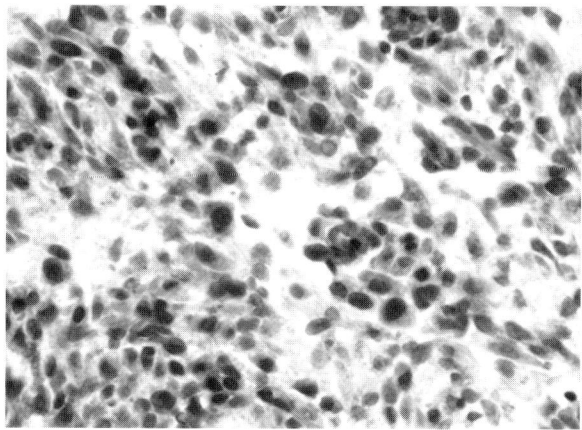

Fig. 3. Antibodies directed against Epstein-Barr virus demonstrate viral infection in inflammatory pseudotumors, as seen in this figure. There is strong nuclear staining of virtually all cells in the proliferation.

genesis of some angiocentric lymphomas and in these cases, staining with LMP may be helpful in confirming a diagnosis and in understanding its pathogenesis. Post-transplant lymphoproliferative disorders may also be EBV induced and these, too, can be confirmed with immunostains directed against EBV *(13)*. Oral hairy leukoplakia is caused, in part, by EBV infection and the virus can be detected in these cases. EBV is also implicated in the pathogenesis of inflammatory pseudotumors (Fig. 3) *(14)*.

A molecule that cross-reacts with LMP-1 antibodies has been described in benign and malignant melanocytic proliferations. Polymerase chain reaction (PCR) technology has demonstrated, however, that this protein is not related directly to EBV and such staining should not be misconstrued as viral infection in the skin *(15)*.

Technical Considerations

Antibodies directed against the LMP-1 portion of the EBV are widely available and work well on routinely processed tissue sections.

Summary

There is little need for most diagnostic dermatopathology laboratories to stock antibodies directed against EBV. These viruses only rarely are implicated in cutaneous diseases.

Spirochetes

Introduction

Warthin-Starry and other silver stains are notoriously difficult to interpret within the skin. This is partially because of all of the elastic tissue and melanin, both of which precipitate silver in this stains. Recently, antibodies directed against spirochetal antigens have been developed, with limited success. Some authors have described antibodies specific for Borrelia burgdorferi and have claimed complete specificity. These authors found no cross-reactivity of their antibody with Treponema pallidum *(16)*. However, this antibody has not yet become widely available.

Other antibodies directed against Treponema pallidum have been developed and used with some degree of efficacy *(17)*.

Diagnostic Utility

Anti-borrelia burgdorferi antibodies can be useful in making a diagnosis of erythema chronicum migrans (associated with Lyme disease). European authors have also found the antibody helpful in confirming the etiologies in cases of morphea, lymphocytoma, and lichen sclerosis and acrodermatitis chronica atrophicans *(16,18)*. American authors have not shared this experience.

Anti-Treponema pallidum antibodies used with a standard avidin-biotin-immunoperoxidase technique have been shown to be more sensitive at detecting organisms within skin specimens than darkfield examinations and other techniques *(17,19)*.

Technical Considerations

Anti-spirochetal antibodies are still not widely available and provide variable results. Commercial products are available that work on routinely processed tissue. It is likely that over time these reagents will become more sensitive and specific and will attain wider circulation.

Summary

There is not yet a widespread experience with these antibodies. Given the difficulty in interpreting Warthin-Starry (or other silver-based) stains when looking for rare spirochetes, there is great promise that such antibodies will be a welcome tool for the diagnostic dermatopathology laboratory.

Mycobacteria

Introduction

Polyclonal antibodies directed against Mycobacteria bovis (BCG) have been developed for use in diagnostic immunopathology.

Diagnostic Utility

Anti-BCG antibodies label a wide range of bacteria, including mycobacteria and fungi with little specificity. Atypical mycobacteria and sporotrichosis are also recognized by these antibodies *(20)*. They do not recognize spirochetes and protozoa such as leishmania *(21)*. Anti-BCG antibodies have proven especially helpful in diagnosing cases of indeterminate and borderline leprosy. In these cases, histochemical stains reveal organisms in only about 30% of cases, while immunostaining found organisms in 50–60% of cases examined *(22–24)*.

Technical Considerations

The anti-BCG antibodies that are commercially available work very well in formalin-fixed, paraffin-embedded tissue sections. The staining is relatively strong with little background staining. No antigen retrieval pretreatment is ordinarily necessary.

Summary

The anti-BCG antibody is very useful as a screen for infectious processes. It stains most bacteria including mycobacteria and most fungi, including sporotrichosis. It does not stain spirochetes or protozoa. Thus, as a screening tool, the antibody is very useful. However, there is absolutely no specificity to a positive result, so a diagnosis of a precise infectious process cannot be made based upon a positive staining reaction. Therefore, this antibody serves a useful, but somewhat limited role in diagnostic dermatopathology.

Rickettsiae

Summary

Antibodies directed against Rickettsia rickettsii are commercially available. These antibodies have been shown to be very sensitive in detecting organisms in endothelial cells in biopsies of infected skin *(25)*. Direct immunofluorescence demonstrated no advantage over immunoperoxidase on formalin-fixed, paraffin-embedded tissue sections for identifying organisms in several studies *(26,27)*.

Antibodies directed against Rickettsia akari also have been shown to work with great sensitivity. This organism gives rise to rickettsialpox. Antibodies directed against the offending organism have been effectively localized to macrophages in infected individuals. The immunoperoxidase technique proved more sensitive than a direct immunofluorescence procedure in this population *(28)*. These antibodies have not yet received widespread usage and it is difficult to assess the efficacy of them at this time.

References

1. Worrell, J. T. and Cockerell, C. J. (1997) Histopathology of periperal nerves in cutaneous herpesvirus infection. *Am. J. Dermatopathol.* **19**, 133–137.
2. Lee, J. Y. and Peel, R. (1989) Concurrent cytomegalovirus and herpes simplex virus infections in skin biopsy specimens from two AIDS patients with fatal CMV infection. *Am. J. Dermatopathol.* **11**, 136–143.
3. Volpi, A., Lakeman, A. D., Pereira, L., and Stagno, S. (1983) Monoclonal antibodies for rapid diagnosis and typing of genital herpes infections during pregnancy. *Am. J. Obstet. Gynecol.* **146**, 813–815.
4. Solomon, A. R. (1988) New diagnostic tests for herpes simplex and varicella zoster infectoins. *J. Am. Acad. Dermatol.* **18**, 218–221.
5. Nikkels, A. F., Debrus, S., Sadzot-Delvaux, C., Piette, J., Delvenne, P., Rentier, B., and Pierard, G. E. (1993) Comparative immunohistochemical study of herpes simplex and varicella-zoster infections. *Vircows. Arch. A. Pathol. Anat. Histopathol.* **422**, 121–126.
6. Fouchard, N., Lacoste, V., Couppie, P., Develoux, M., Mauclere, P., Michel, P., et al. (2000) Detection and genetic polymorphism of human herpes virus type 8 in endemic or epidemic Kaposi's sarcoma from West and Central Africa, and South America. *Int. J. Cancer.* **85**, 166–170.
7. Nuovo, M. and Nuovo, G. (2001) Utility of HHV8 RNA detection for differentiating Kaposi's sarcoma from its mimics. *J. Cutan. Pathol.* **28**, 248–255.
8. Smoller, B. R., Chang, P. P., and Kamel, O. W. (1997) No role for human herpes virus 8 in the etiology of infantile capillary hemangioma. *Mod. Pathol.* **10**, 675–678.
9. Maiorana, A., Luppi, M., Barozzi, P., Collina, G., Fano, R. A., and Torelli, G. (1997) Detection of human herpes virus type 8 DNA sequences as a valuable aid in the differential diagnosis of Kaposi's sarcoma. *Mod. Pathol.* **10**, 182–187.
10. Sumiyoshi, Y., akashi, K., and Kikuchi, M. (1994) Detection of human herpes virus 6 (HHV6) in the skin of a patient with primary HHV6 infection and erythroderma. *J. Clin. Pathol.* **47**, 762–763.
11. Horn, T. D., Farmer, E. R., Vogelsang, G. B., Wingard, J. R., and Santos, G. W. (1989) Cutaneous graft-vs-host reaction lacks evidence of cutaneous cytomegalovirus by the immunoperoxidase technique. *J. Invest. Dermatol.* **93**, 92–95.
12. Nico, M. M., Cymbalista, N. C., Hurtado, Y. C., and Borges, L. H. (2000) Perianal cytomegalovirus ulcer in an HIV infected patient: case report and review of the literature. *J. Dermatol.* **27**, 99–105.

13. Chai, C., White, W. L., Shea, C. R., and Prieto, V. G. (1999) Epstein Barr virus-associated lymphoproliferative-disorders primarily involving the skin. *J. Cutan. Pathol.* **26,** 242–247.
14. Gulley, M. L. (2001) Molecular diagnosis of Epstein-Barr virus-related diseases. *J. Mol. Diagn.* **3,** 1–10.
15. Bertalot, G., Biasi, M. O., Gramegna, M., Askaa, J., Dell'Orto, P., and Viale, G. (2000) Immunoreactivity for latent membrane protein 1 of Epstein-Barr virus in nevi and melanomas is not related to the viral infection. *Virchows Arch.* **436,** 553–559.
16. Arrese Estrada, J., Melote, P., Hermanns, J. F., and Pierard, G. E. (1991) Immunohistochemistry of Borrelia type spirochetes. *Ann. Dermaol. Venereol.* **118,** 277–279.
17. Lee, W. S., Lee, M. G., Chung, K. Y., and Lee, J. B. (1991) Detection of Treponema pallidum in tissue: a comparative study of the avidin-biotin-peroxidase complex, indirect immunoperoxidase, FTA-ABS complement techniques and the darkfield method. *Yonsei Med. J.* **32,** 335–341.
18. Aberer, E. and Stanek, G. (1987) Histological evidence for spirochetal origin of morphea and lichen sclerosus et atrophicans. *Am. J. Dermatopathol.* **9,** 374–379.
19. Chung, K. Y., Lee, M. G., Chon, C. Y., and Lee, J. B. (1989) Syphilitic gastritis: demonstration of Treponema pallidum with the use of fluorescent treponemal antibody absorption complement and immunoperoxidase stains. *J. Am. Acad. Dermatol.* **21,** 183–185.
20. Byrd, J., Mehregan, D. R., and Mehregan, D. A. (2001) Utility of anti-bacillus Calmette-Guerin antibodies as a screen for organisms in sporotrichoid infections. *J. Am. Acad. Dermatol.* **44,** 261–264.
21. Bonenberger, T. E., Ihrke, P. J., Naydan, D. K., and Affolter, V. K. (2001) Rapid identification of tissue micro-organisms in skin biopsy specimens from domestic animals using polyclonal BCG antibody. *Vet. Dermatol.* **12,** 41–47.
22. Natrajan, M., Katoch, K., Katoch, V. M., and Bharadwaj, V. P. (1995) Enhancement in the histological diagnosis of indeterminate leprosy by demonstration of mycobacterial antigens. *Acta Leprol.* **9,** 201–207.
23. Barbosa Junior, A., Silva, T. C., Patel, B. N., Santos, M. I., Wakamatsu, A., and Alves, V. A. (1994) Demonstration of mycobacterial antigens in skin biopsies form suspected leprosy cases in the absence of bacilli. *Pathol. Res. Pract.* **190,** 782–785.
24. Mshana, R. N., Humber, D. P., Harboe, M., and Belehu, A. (1983) Demonstration of mycobacterial antigens in nerve biopsies from leprosy patients using peroxidase-antiperoxidase immunoenzyme technique. *Clin. Immunol. Immunopathol.* **29,** 359–368.
25. Kao, G. F., Evancho, C. D., Ioffe, O., Lowitt, M. H., and Dumler, J. S. (1997) Cutaneous histopathology of Rocky Mountain spotted fever. *J. Cutan. Pathol.* **24,** 604–610.
26. Procop, G. W., Burchette, J. L., Jr., Howell, D. N., and Sexton, D. J. (1997) Immunoperoxidase and immunofluorescent staining of Rickettsia rickettsii in skin biopsies. A comparative study. *Arch. Pathol. Lab.* **121,** 894–899.
27. White, W. L., Patrick, J. D., and Miller, L. R. (1994) Evaluation of immunoperoxidase techniques to detect Rickettsia rickettsii in fixed tissue sections. *Am. J. Clin. Pathol.* **101,** 747–752.
28. Walker, D. H., Hudnall, S. D., Szaniawski, W. K., and Feng, H. M. (1999) Monoclonal antibody-based immunohistochemical diagnosis of rickettsialpox: the macrophage is the principal target. *Mod. Pathol.* **12,** 529–533.

9 Markers Useful in Detecting Metastatic Disease

Metastases to the skin are encountered with some frequency in diagnostic dermatopathology. They occur in from 0.7–9% of all patients with cancer *(1)*. In many cases, there is a known primary site for the metastatic lesion. In these cases, routine histologic sections may provide enough evidence to label a metastatic tumor as likely arising from the known primary source. In some cases, however, routine sections may not be diagnostic, or the source of the primary neoplasm may not be known.

Cutaneous metastases may be the presenting sign of disease *(1)*. In these cases, it can be helpful to be aware of some antibodies that are not ordinarily associated with cutaneous cell types, but are found in tumor cells that may spread to the skin. In this chapter, I will briefly present a few of the more specific antibodies associated with neoplasms that may metastasize to the skin *(2)*.

It is important to realize that antibodies commonly associated with breast carcinoma, the most frequently encountered cutaneous metastases, are also invariably associated with eccrine neoplasms and are addressed in Chapter 3. At this point, there is not a reliable method to immunophenotypically distinguish between a primary eccrine neoplasm and a metastatic lesion from the breast. Though there is not yet any published literature to this effect, differential expression of Her-2-neu (expressed by metastatic breast carcinomas, but not by eccrine neoplasms) may prove to be helpful making this distinction.

Prostate Specific Antigen/Prostatic Acid Phosphatase
Introduction

Prostate specific antigen is a 30 kD serine protease with unknown physiologic function *(3)*. Prostatic acid phosphatase is a phospho-tyrosyl-protein phosphatase *(4)*. Monoclonal antibodies directed

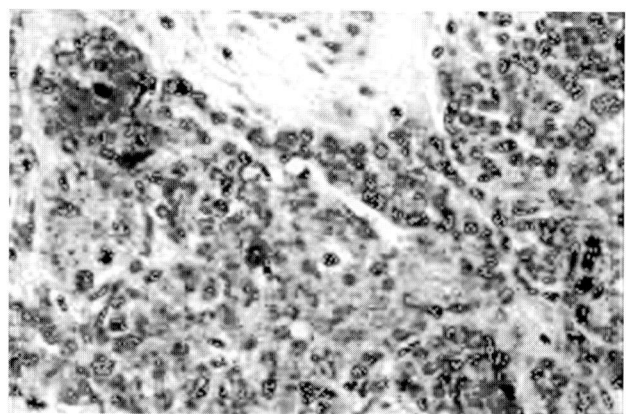

Fig. 1. Epithelium in adenocarcinoma from the prostate strongly expresses prostate specific antigen.

against these proteins have attained widespread use in surgical pathology.

Diagnostic Utility

Cutaneous metastases from prostate adenocarcinomas are quite uncommon. However, they do occur and can be the presenting manifestation of the disease. In these cases, the patient presents with a tumor nodule that has the histologic features of an adenocarcinoma within the dermis. Should prostate carcinoma be in the differential diagnosis, immunostains for prostate specific antigen and prostatic acid phosphatase provide more specific information than do other markers for adenocarcinoma (such as CEA) (Fig. 1) (2,5). The literature offers mixed results as to which of the two markers is more sensitive (6). There is no extensive study in the literature that suggests sensitivities or specificities for these markers in detecting cutaneous lesions of metastatic prostate carcinoma. This is probably due, at least in part, to the rarity of this presentation.

Rare neoplasms other than prostatic adenocarcinomas have been shown to express prostate specific antigen. This antigen has been seen in a single salivary gland tumor that was negative when stained with prostatic acid phosphatase (3). Primary breast carcinomas in males can also express prostate specific antigen (7).

Technical Considerations

Antibodies directed against prostate specific antigen and prostatic acid phosphatase are commercially available. They work well on routinely fixed tissue sections and do not ordinarily require any special pretreatment. However, HIER has been shown to augment the staining intensity with these antibodies *(8)*.

Summary

As is the case with all antibodies in this chapter, there is no primary cutaneous disease recognized by prostate specific antigen or prostatic acid phosphatase. These markers may be useful in the work-up of a metastatic tumor with no known primary source, but unless the laboratory volume is quite high, this scenario is not likely to be frequent enough to warrant stocking these antibodies.

Thyroid Stimulating Hormone

Introduction

Thyroglobulin is a protein that is produced by the thyroid gland. It is believed to be essentially specific for this organ.

Diagnostic Utility

Thyroglobulin antibodies have been shown to be relatively specific for thyroid neoplasms *(2,5)*. In a small series, this antibody proved to be 100% specific and 100% sensitive for metastatic thyroid carcinomas *(9)*. However, as is the case with any antibody, these results should be interpreted with caution, as only a small series of cases was examined. Positive staining with anti-thyroglobulin antibodies has proven to be useful in confirming cutaneous metastases from follicular and papillary thyroid neoplasms *(10–13)*. It is also known that medullary carcinomas of the thyroid express thyroglobulin in a minority of cases *(14)*, The thyroidal component of struma ovarii expresses thyroglobulin *(15)*.

Technical Considerations

Anti-thyroglobulin antibodies are commercially available. They work well in routinely fixed tissue and do not require any pretreatment. Cytoplasmic staining is strong and diffuse in most cases. HIER has been shown to increase staining intensity *(8)*.

Summary

Anti-thyroglobulin antibodies are generally not important in diagnostic dermatopathology. While highly specific and sensitive, cutaneous metastases from thyroid malignancies are very rare.

Thyroid Transcription Factor-1 (TTF-1)

Introduction

Thyroid transcription factor-1 is one of three such factors present in thyroid follicular cells. It appears to play some role in the differentiation of these cells and in their ability to produce thyroid hormone (16). The same protein has also been found in pulmonary epithelial cells (17).

Diagnostic Utility

TTF-1 is thought to be relatively specific for neoplasms of thyroid origin (2). However, this is not absolute. TTF-1 expression has also been demonstrated in sclerosing hemangiomas of the lung (17).

Perhaps the most common usage for anti-TTF-1 in dermatopathology at this point is in making the distinction between Merkel cell carcinomas and metastatic small cell carcinomas of the lung. TTF-1 is not expressed by Merkel cell carcinomas (18,19). In contrast, TTF-1 is strongly expressed by the vast majority of metastatic small cell carcinomas of the lung (18,19). TTF-1 is also expressed by other types of small cell carcinoma that arise from extrapulmonary sources (20).

Technical Considerations

Anti-TTF-1 antibodies are commercially available. They provide reproducibly strong staining on routinely processed tissue sections.

Summary

As is the case with the other antibodies discussed in this chapter, there is little need for this antibody on a routine, daily basis in diagnostic dermatopathology. It may be helpful in distinguishing Merkel cell carcinomas from metastatic small cell carcinomas, and in defining a metastatic tumor as being from the thyroid gland, but these situations are unlikely to arise on a regular basis in most laboratories.

Miscellaneous Tumor Markers

Summary

Antibodies directed against alpha-fetoprotein, human chorionic gonadotropism and CA125 have all proven to be useful markers in surgical pathology. The antigens recognized by these antibodies have limited patterns of expression. Thus, detection of expression of one or more of these antibodies is useful in narrowing down the origin of an unknown primary tumor. However, as none of the tumors that express these antigens commonly gives rise to cutaneous metastases, it is not cost-effective for these reagents to be readily available in most dermatopathology laboratories.

Sex Hormone Receptors

Estrogen, progesterone, and androgen receptors are discussed in Chapter 3.

References

1. Schwartz, R. A. (1995) Cutaneous metastatic disease. *J. Am. Acad. Dermatol.* **33**, 161–182.
2. Hammar, S. P. (1998) Metastatic adenocarcinoma of unknown primary origin. *Hum. Pathol.* **29**, 1393–1402.
3. James, G. K., Pudek, M., Berean, K.W., Diamandis, E.P., and Archibald, B.L. (1996) Salivary duct carcinoma secreting prostate-specific antigen. *Am. J. Clin. Pathol.* **106**, 242–247.
4. Chu, T. M. (1990) Prostate cancer-associated markers. *Immunol. Ser.* **53**, 339–356.
5. Brown, R. W., Campagna, L. B., Dunn, J. K., and Cagle, P. T. (1997) Immunohistochemical identification of tumor markers in metastatic adenocarcinoma. A diagnostic adjunct in the determination of primary site. *Am. J. Clin. Pathol.* **107**, 12–19.
6. Cho, K. R. and Epstein, J. I. (1987) Metastatic prostate carcinoma to supradiaphragmatic lymph nodes. A clinicopathologic and immunohistochemical study. *Am. J. Surg. Pathol.* **11**, 457–463.
7. Gupta, R. K. (1999) Immunoreactivity of prostate-specific antigen in male breast carcinomas: two examples of a diagnostic pitfall in discriminating a primary breast cancer from metastatic prostate carcinoma. *Diagn. Cytopathol.* **21**, 167–169.
8. Gown, A. M., de Wever, N., and Battifora, H. (1993) Microwave-based antigenic unmasking. A revolutionary new technique for routine immunohistochemistry. *Appl. Immunohistochem.* **1**, 256–266.
9. de Almeida, P. C. and Pestana, C. B. (1989) Use of immunohistochemistry in detecting the primary site in neoplasm metastasis. AMB. *Rev. Assoc. Med. Bras.* **35**, 84–87.

10. Rico, M. J. and Penneys, N. S. (1985) Metastatic follicular carcinoma of the thyroid to the skin: a case confirmed by immunohistochemistry. *J. Cutan. Pathol.* **12,** 103–105.
11. Gal, R., Aranof, A., Gertzmann, H., and Kessler, E. (1987) The potential value of the demonstration of thyroglobulin by immunoperoxidase techniques in fine needle aspiration cytology. *Acta. Cytol.* **31,** 713–716.
12. Koller, E. A., Tourtelot, J. B., Pak, H. S., Cobb, M. W., Moad, J. C., and Flynn, E. A. (1998) Papillary and follicular thyroid carcinoma metastatic to the skin: a case report and review of the literature. *Thyroid* **8,** 1045–1050.
13. Lissak, B., Vannetzel, J. M., Gallouedec, N., Berrod, J. L., and Rieu, M. (1995) Solitary skin metastasis as the presenting feature of differentiated thyroid microcarcinoma: report of two cases. *J. Endocrinol. Invest.* **18,** 813–816.
14. Uribe, M., Fenoglio-Preiser, C. M., Grimes, M., and Feind, C. (1985) Medullary carcinoma of the thyroid gland. Clinical, pathological, and immunohistochemical features with review of the literature. *Am. J. Surg. Pathol.* **9,** 577–594.
15. Gould, S. F., Lopez, R. L., and Speers, W. C. (1983) Malignant struma ovarii. A case report and literature review. *J. Reprod .Med.* **28,** 415–419.
16. Damante, G., Tell, G., and Di Lauro, R. (2001) A unique combination of transcription factors controls differentiation of thyroid cells. *Prog. Nucleic. Acid. Res. Mol. Biol.* **66,** 307–356.
17. Illei, P. B., Rosai, J., and Klimstra, D. S. (2001) Expression of thyroid transcription factor-1 and other markers in sclerosing hemangioma of the lung. *Arch. Pathol. Lab. Med.* **125,** 1335–1339.
18. Hanly, A. J., Elgart, G. W., Jorda, M., Smith, J., and Nadji, M. (2000) Analysis of thyroid transcription factor-1 ad cytokeratin 20 separates merkel cell carcinoma from small cell carcinoma of the lung. *J. Cutan. Pathol.* **27,** 118–120.
19. Leech, S. N., Kolar, A. J., Barrett, P. D., Sinclair, S. A., and Leonard, N. (2001) Merkel cell carcinoma can be distinguished from metastatic small cell carcinoma using antibodies to cytokeratin 20 and thyroid transcription factor 1. *J. Clin. Pathol.* **54,** 727–729.
20. Cheuk, W., Kwan, M. Y., Suster, S., and Chan, J. K. (2001) Immunostaining for thyroid transcription factor 1 and cytokeratin 20 aids the distinction of small cell carcinoma from Merkel cell carcinoma, but not pulmonary from extrapulmonary small cell carcinomas. *Arch. Pathol. Lab. Med.* **125,** 228–231.

III VIGNETTES

10 Vignettes

Introduction

The final section of this volume is a series of vignettes designed to provide representative examples of the concepts put forth in the earlier sections of the book. For each case, a representative clinical history is presented along with actual routinely processed biopsy material. In many cases, the biopsy specimens are sub-optimal, adding to the difficulties in arriving at a diagnosis. These cases were selected in order to exemplify the real-life situations that diagnostic dermatopathologists find themselves encountering. In each case, a differential diagnosis is presented based upon the biopsy findings and an immunostaining strategy is presented in tabular form. The tables are over-simplified, presenting expected immunostaining results as "+" or "−" for situations where a positive result is expected in >75% or <5% of cases, respectively. Less reproducible situations are explained more completely in the table. I chose to present the data this way so that the tables could serve as quick and useful references; however, it is absolutely essential to recognize that the "+" and "−" designations are not absolute. For more precise percentages, the reader is strongly advised to refer back to the appropriate chapters, earlier in the book and the cited references. A photographic depiction of the staining results is presented following the tabular data. Again, readers are encouraged to return to the main sections of the text for the best references.

Vignette A

Differential Diagnosis of Intraepidermal, Atypical Pagetoid Cells

The patient is a 67-yr-old woman with who presented with an erythematous, scaly plaque on her vulva that she described as being intensely pruritic. On clinical examination, the lesion appeared erythematous and slightly hyperpigmented. The clinical differential diagnosis included extra-mammary Paget's disease, squamous cell carcinoma *in situ*, seborrheic dermatitis, intertrigo, and candidiasis.

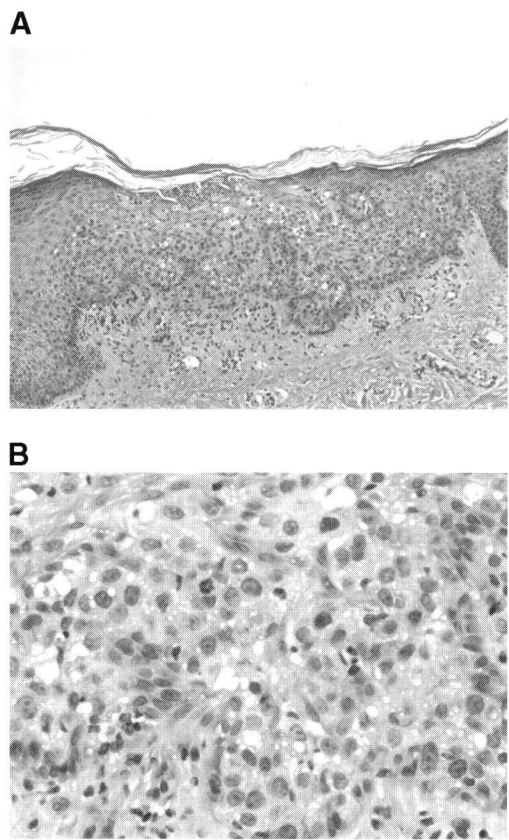

Fig. 1. (A) Low magnification demonstrates an intra-epidermal population of atypical cells. **(B)** Higher magnification demonstrates atypical cells with abundant pale staining cytoplasm.

A small punch biopsy was performed and yielded the following specimen as seen in Fig. 1A,B.

While the clinical presentation was most in keeping with a diagnosis of extramammary Paget's disease, the histology was difficult to interpret and a differential diagnosis was generated. In order to resolve the diagnostic dilemma, a strategy for immunolabeling tissue sections was developed and is presented in Table 1.

The staining pattern is depicted in Fig. 2A–C. As can be seen, there is strong staining of the large, atypical cells with cytokeratin 7 and epithelial membrane antigen. The staining with AE1/AE3 is somewhat difficult to interpret and there is no staining with S100. The negative

Table 1
Differential Diagnosis of Atypical Intraepidermal Cells

	Cytokeratin 7	Epithelial membrane antigen	S100	AE1/AE3
Extramammary Paget's disease	+	+	−	+
Squamous cell carcinoma *in situ*	−	Focal intermittent staining	−	±
Melanoma *in situ*	−	−	+	−

S100 stain provides strong evidence against a diagnosis of melanoma; however, it is imperative that the tissue sections be examined for the presence of positive internal control staining in order to insure adequacy of the test. Cytokeratin 7 expression is expected in Paget's disease and extramammary Paget's disease, making this diagnosis most likely. Cytokeratin 7 expression is not a feature of squamous cell carcinomas. The anti-keratin antibodies and the anti-epithelial membrane antigen are useful in confirming the primary staining results. These antigens can be expressed by keratinocytes in squamous cell carcinomas, but this is an inconstant finding. Cells in extramammary Paget's disease usually express them.

Vignette B

Differential Diagnosis of "Blue Cell Tumors"

A 27-yr-old woman presented to her local dermatologist with a 1 cm tender nodule on her forearm. She claimed it had been there for about 2 mo and was very tender to palpation. Examination revealed a dermal nodule with no overlying epidermal changes. The clinical differential diagnosis included angiolipoma, eccrine spiradenoma, glomus tumor and leiomyoma. A biopsy was performed.

The histologic changes are depicted in Fig. 3A,B. The differential diagnosis included glomus tumor, eccrine spiradenoma, lymphoma, Merkel cell carcinoma and less likely a metastasis, though there was minimal cytologic atypia. An immunostaining strategy was designed and is seen in Table 2.

Highlights from the immunostaining are seen in Fig. 4A–D. As is shown in Fig. 4A, glomus tumors stain strongly with anti-smooth

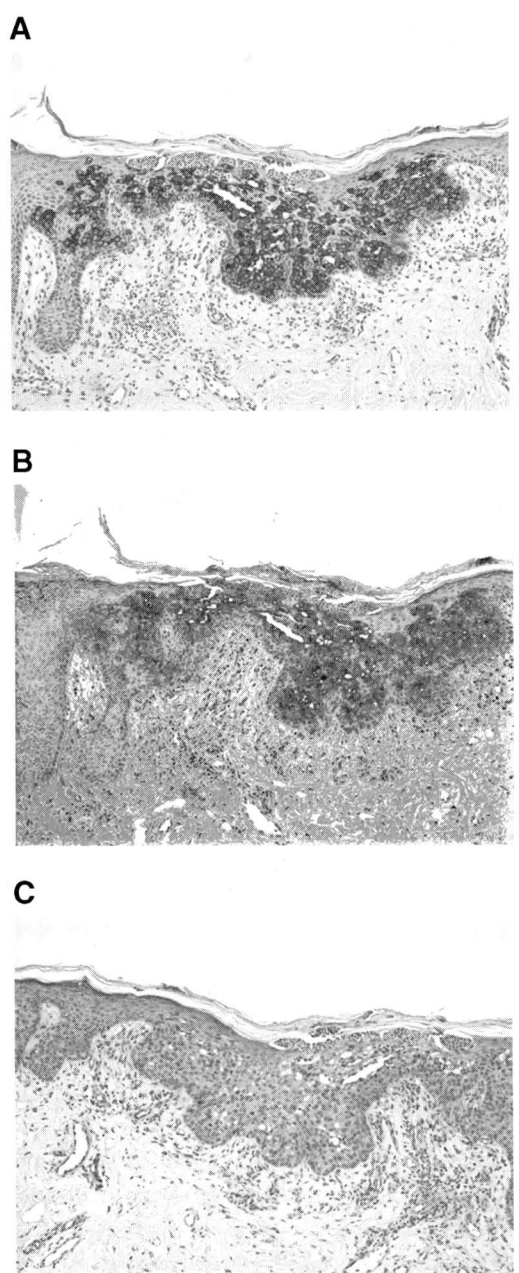

Fig. 2. (A) Anti-cytokeratin 7 is strongly expressed by the atypical cells within the epidermis, but not by the background keratinocytes. **(B)** Similarly, anti-EMA labels the tumor cells but not the background keratinocytes within the epidermis.**(C)** Anti-S100 does not label the intraepidermal tumor cells.

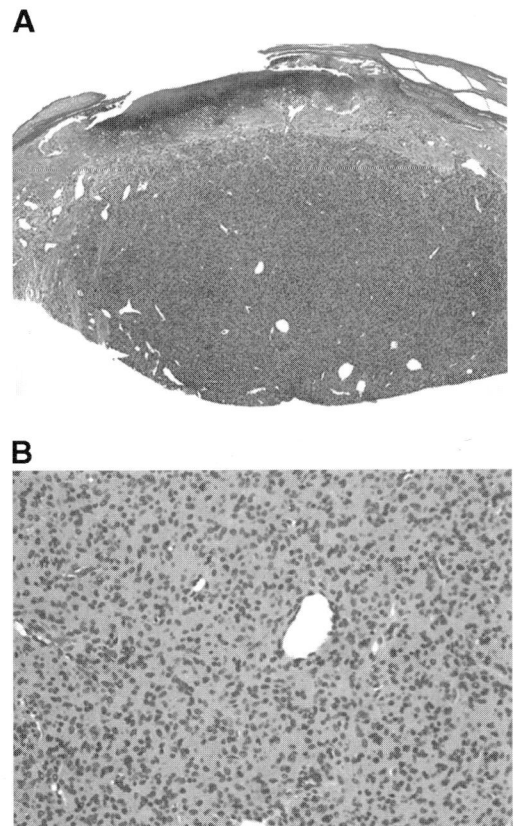

Fig. 3. (A) Low power demonstrates a well-circumscribed dermal nodule comprised of small, dark cells. **(B)** The tumor cells are remarkably uniform with minimal cytologic atypia.

Table 2
Differential Diagnosis to Small Blue Cell Tumors in the Dermis

	Smooth muscle actin	CD3	CD20	CK cocktail	CK 20	CK 7
Glomus tumor	+	−	−	−	−	−
Lymphoma	−	+/−	+/−	−	−	−
Eccrine spiradenoma	−	−	−	+	−	+ (focal)
Merkel cell Carcinoma	−	−	−	+	+	−
Metastatic carcinoma	−	−	−	+	−	+/−

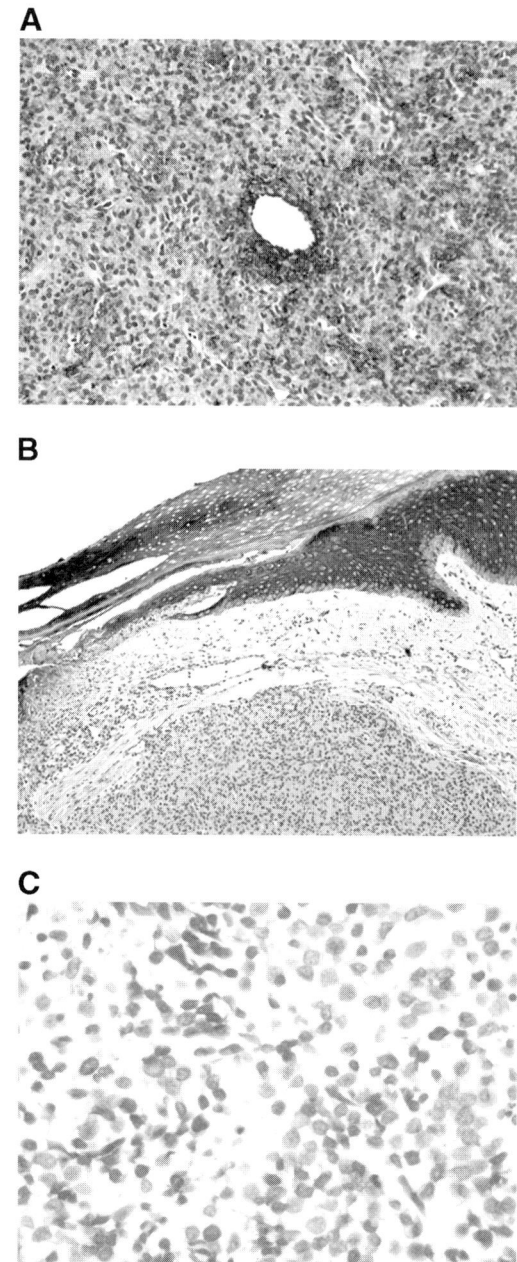

Fig. 4. (A) Anti-smooth muscle actin strongly stains the tumor cells. **(B)** AE1/ AE3 anti-cytokeratin cocktail does not stain the tumor cells. **(C)** Anti-CD3 does not recognize the tumor cells.

muscle actin, being neoplasms of modified smooth muscle cells. Note that we used a combination of anti-CD3 and anti-CD20 to rule out the possibility of lymphoma in this case. Alternatively, we could have used an anti-leukocyte common antigen antibody for this purpose. (We do not currently stock anti-LCA, as we find little use for it in our routine practice of dermatopathology). Anti-cytokeratin cocktails are not able to discriminate between eccrine neoplasms and metastatic carcinomas, as both would likely be focally positive. It is possible that the anti-cytokeratin 7 antibody might be helpful. It labels eccrine ductular differentiation, but some carcinomas will also stain with this marker (*see* Chapter 3). Thus, it may not be possible to make this distinction with immunostains. Routine histologic findings, however, are helpful in that cytologic atypia is not a feature of eccrine spiradenoma. Merkel cell carcinomas may also be positive with anti-keratin cocktails, but usually express cytokeratin 20 and not cytokeratin 7, in contrast to eccrine neoplasms. Expression of smooth muscle actin is unique to glomus cell tumors in this differential diagnosis.

Vignette C

Differential Diagnosis of Densely Cellular Spindle Cell Tumor

A 70-yr-old man presented with a slightly hyperpigmented nodule on his hand that had been growing slowly for the past 3–4 mo. It was not painful and he was otherwise in good health. The nodule was firm and had no overlying surface changes. The clinical differential diagnosis included dermatofibroma, dermatofibrosarcoma protuberans, Kaposi's sarcoma and a foreign body giant cell granulomatous reaction. A biopsy was performed and is represented in Fig. 5A,B.

The histologic differential diagnosis included mainly Kaposi's sarcoma, based upon the extravasation of erythrocytes, and dermatofibrosarcoma protuberans, based upon the dense cellularity with minimal pleomorphism or cytologic atypia. Also considered were spindle cell melanoma and a solitary fibrous tumor (which was thought to be extremely unlikely). An immunostaining panel was developed to resolve this diagnostic dilemma and is shown in Table 3.

As is seen in Fig. 6A,B, the tumor cells stained strongly with both anti-CD34 and anti-CD31. They failed to express S100 protein (not

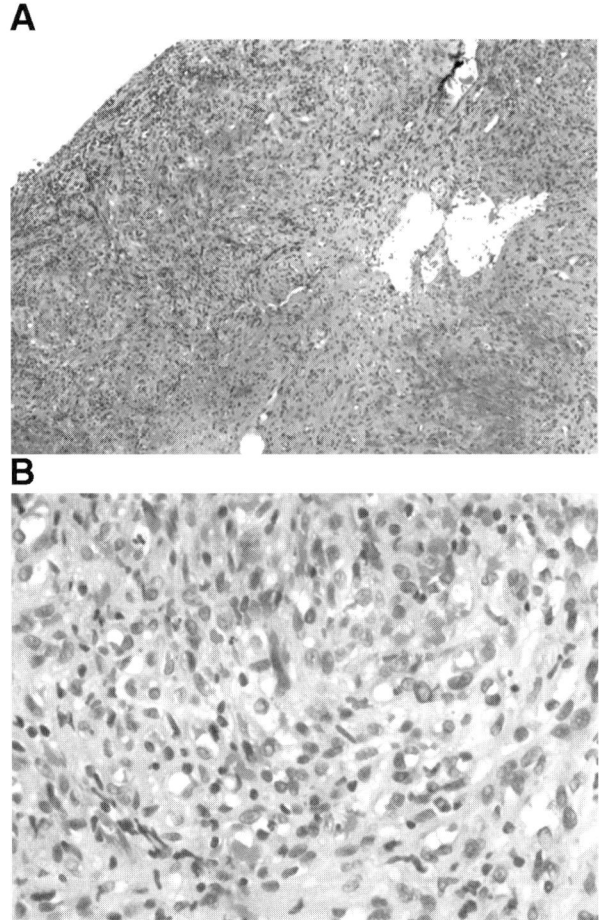

Fig. 5. (A) Low power demonstrates a dermal spindle cell neoplasm with no obvious connection to the epidermis. **(B)** Higher magnification reveals a relatively uniform population of spindle shaped cells. There is some extravasation of erythrocytes present within the tumor mass.

Table 3
Differential Diagnosis to Dermal Spindle Cell Neoplasm

	CD31	CD34	S100
Kaposi's sarcoma	+	+	−
Melanoma	−	−	+
Dermatofibrosarcoma protuberans	−	+	−
Solitary fibrous tumor	−	+	−

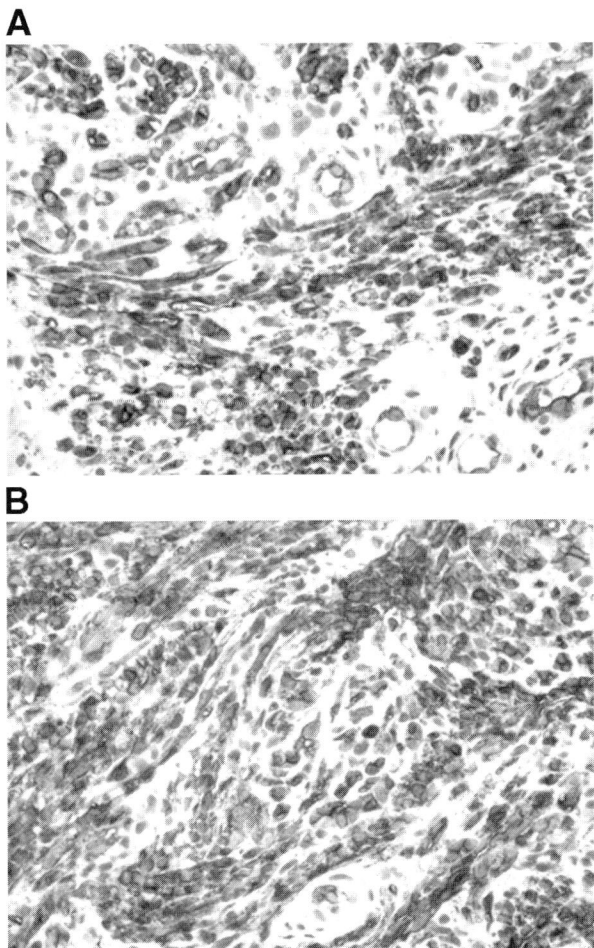

Fig. 6. (A) CD31 is strongly expressed by the spindle cells. **(B)** The spindle cells also strongly express CD34.

shown). The important things to note in this work-up is that demonstration of CD34 alone would not have been sufficient. Three of the four major entities in the differential diagnosis are known to express CD34 strongly and diffusely. Only a spindle cell melanoma would have been excluded based upon the finding of CD34 positivity. CD31 is a much more specific antibody, helping to identify the cellular component of the tumor as being of endothelial cell origin. While endothelial cells express CD34, a wide range of other cell types also expresses it.

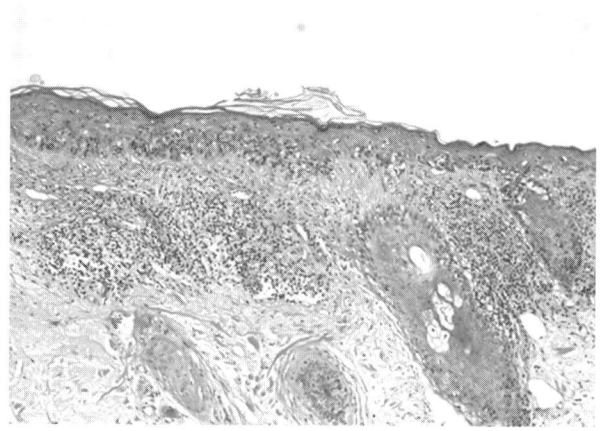

Fig. 7. Histologic sections demonstrate an atrophic epidermis with atypical basaloid cells.

It might also be noted that the staining profile of dermatofibrosarcoma protuberans and solitary fibrous tumors is identical with this antibody panel. In fact, they are very difficult to distinguish using immunopathologic techniques. Examination of routine histologic features and clinical presentation remain the best ways to differentiate these two entities.

It is also essential to note that anti-S100 antibodies are the appropriate probes to exclude melanoma. For all subtypes of melanoma, anti-S100 is the most sensitive marker. This is especially true of spindle cell melanomas that only rarely express MART-1, HMB-45, or tyrosinase.

Vignette D

Differential Diagnosis of Actinic Keratosis vs Lentigo Maligna

A 77-yr-old man was evaluated by his dermatologist and found to have a macular, irregular hyperpigmented patch on his face. He had extensive sun damage and a history of many previous actinic keratoses and basal cell carcinomas. The clinical differential diagnosis included pigmented actinic keratosis, solar lentigo and lentigo maligna type of melanoma *in situ*. Biopsies were performed and are depicted in Fig. 7.

Table 4
Differential Diagnosis of Actinic Keratosis and Lentigo Maligna

	AE1/AE3	S100	MART-1
Actinic keratosis	±	−	−
Lentigo maligna	−	+	+

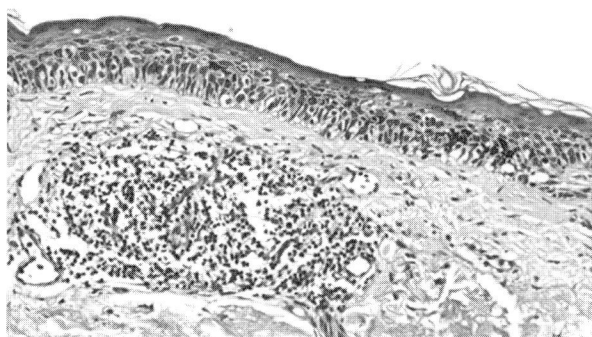

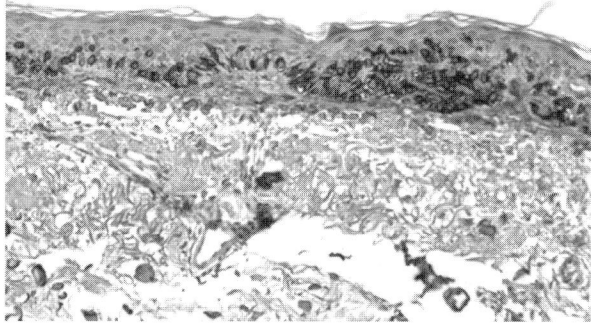

Fig. 8. (A) The atypical cells along the basal layer fail to express cytokeratins recognized by AE1/AE3. (B) Increased numbers of atypical basaloid cells strongly express MART-1, proving that they are melanocytes.

It was difficult, if not impossible, to determine if the atypical cells along the dermal epidermal junction were keratinocytes or melanocytes. A simple immunostaining pattern was created to resolve this simple question. It is presented in Table 4.

Results of the immunostaining are seen in Figs. 8A,B. In cases where the atypical cells are keratinocytes, AE1 may or not be positive. The diagnosis of actinic keratosis can be made with positive staining, but many atypical squamoproliferative processes only focally express the cytokeratins recognized by this antibody. Alternatively, definitive staining of the intraepidermal atypical cells with S100 and/or MART-1 is evidence strongly supportive of a melanoma *in situ*. There is no known cross-reactivity of these antibodies with keratinocytes. Thus, the atypical cells are melanocytes, and in this pattern, represent a melanoma *in situ*. I usually use both antibodies in order to maximize sensitivity. Performance of anti-S100 antibodies may be affected by variations in fixation procedures.

Vignette E

Differential Diagnosis of Cutaneous Lymphoid Infiltrate

A 61-yr-old woman presented to her dermatologist with an erythematous 2 cm nodule on her forehead. There were no epidermal changes and the nodule was firm to palpation. The clinical differential diagnosis included cutaneous lymphoma, lymphocytoma cutis (reactive lymphoid hyperplasia), granuloma annulare and Jessner's lymphocytic infiltrate. A biopsy was performed and revealed the histologic changes seen in Fig. 9A,B.

The histologic differential diagnosis included lymphoma cutis (probable B cell type), Jessner's lymphocytic infiltrate, and cutaneous lymphoid hyperplasia. A panel of antibodies designed to resolve this dilemma was created and is seen in Table 5.

The results of the immunostaining are seen in Fig. 10A–D. Unlike many of the other vignettes presented, staining pattern is essential in making the diagnosis. In cutaneous lymphoid hyperplasia, the dermis is filled with lymphocytes. Germinal centers (follicular centers) can be identified in many cases, and these are highlighted with use of the CD20 antibody. CD3 stains cells in the surrounding zones, recapitulating the pattern seen in reactive lymph nodes. In contrast, as is seen in this case, large sheets of CD20 positive lymphocytes are seen in B cell lymphomas. T cells may be present, but are not seen in an orga-

A

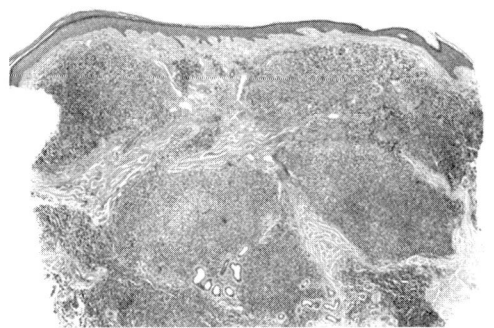

B

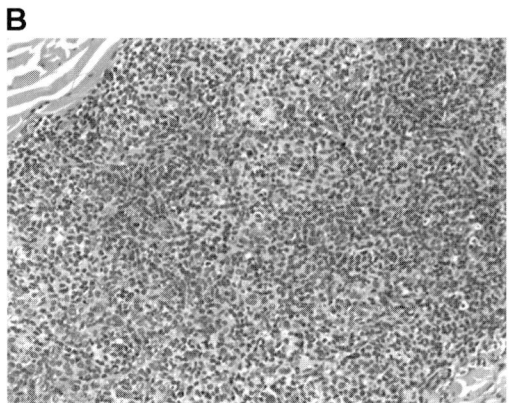

Fig. 9. (A) Low power demonstrates a dense dermal infiltrate of lymphocytes with a prominent Grenz zone. **(B)** Higher magnification reveals a relatively uniform population of lymphocytes, though both small and large cells are seen.

Table 5
Differential Diagnosis of a Dense Dermal Lymphocytic Infiltrate

	CD3	CD20	Kappa light chains	Lambda light chains
Lymphoma	Focal; minority of cells	Sheets of cells	Almost all B cells (or none)	Almost all B cells (or none)
Cutaneous lymphoid hyperplasia	Zones of positive cells	Germinal centers positive	Majority of B cells positive	Minority of B cells positive
Jessner's lymphocytic infiltrate	Diffusely positive	Only rare positive cells	Negative	Negative

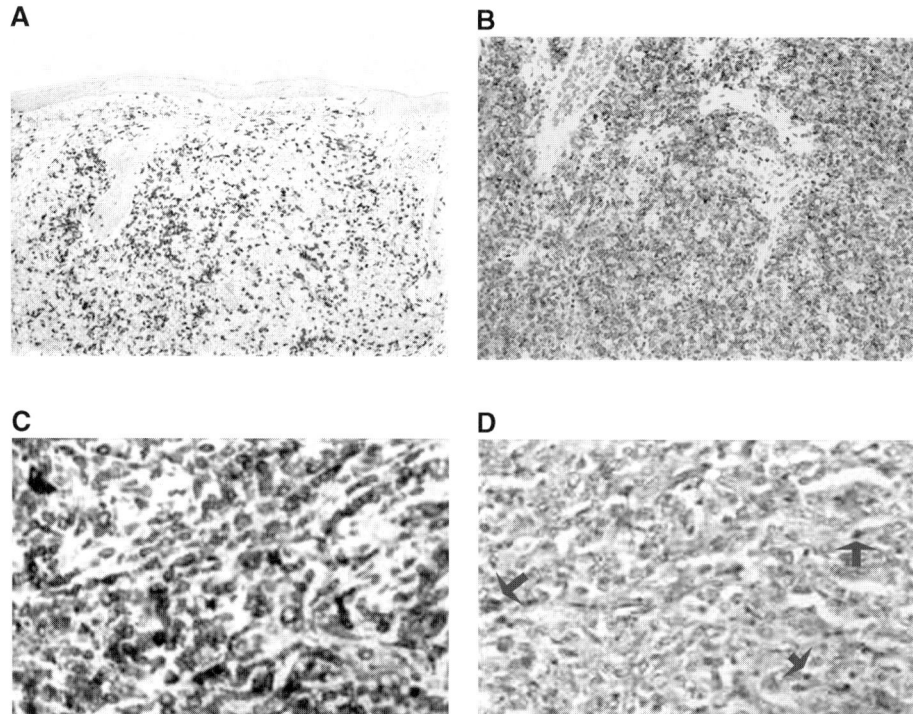

Fig. 10. (A) Anti-CD3 stains only a small number of cells at the periphery of the lymphoid aggregates. **(B)** Sheets of cells express CD20. **(C)** Kappa light chains are expressed by almost all of the CD20 positive cells. **(D)** Expression of lambda light chains is severely restricted in this monoclonal population of neoplastic B cells.

nized pattern around well-formed follicular centers. In this case, strong expression of kappa light chains, and no staining with lambda confirms the monoclonal nature of the infiltrate. The addition of a CD68 antibody may be helpful in highlighting the presence of tingible body macrophages. These cells are found in reactive follicles, but not within neoplastic follicles of follicular center cell B cell lymphomas. I have not found anti-bcl-2 antibodies to be helpful in most cases (*see* Chapter 5).

Jessner's lymphocytic infiltrate is an ill-defined entity that is characterized by a nonepidermotropic, dermal infiltrate of T lymphocytes. Immunostaining such as the panel depicted above would help in making this distinction, as B lymphocytes are present in small numbers scattered throughout the dermis in this process.

Vignette F

Differential Diagnosis of Basal Cell Carcinoma vs Appendageal Neoplasm

A 37-yr-old man presented with a 1 cm nodule on his posterior neck. The tumor had no epidermal changes, was not tender, and was firm and freely mobile. There was an extended clinical differential diagnosis.

The histologic sections are represented in Fig. 11A,B. Abundant ductular or pseudoductules are present admixed with islands of basaloid cells. The characteristic cleft artifact often present in basal cell carcinomas is not present. The differential diagnosis included a basal cell carcinoma and an eccrine epithelioma. An appropriate panel of immunostains was developed and is depicted in Table 6.

The staining results are demonstrated in Fig. 12A–C. There are several important points to underscore with regard to the staining results. First, it should be noted that most basal cell carcinomas do not express the keratins that are detected by cocktails such as CAM 5.2, nor do they produce cytokeratin 7. Thus, it is difficult to find a marker that can reliably be expected to label these neoplasms. (The exception would be that if there is squamatization, the areas with more "squamous" differentiation might express the keratins detected by CAM 5.2 or AE1/AE3. MNF116 is also known to be expressed by basal cell carcinomas.)

Another point to be gleaned from this panel is in the selection of antibodies designed to demonstrate true ductular differentiation. In order to maximize sensitivity, I often will select more than one antibody that potentially labels a certain finding. In this type of case where ductular differentiation might not be so readily found, it is useful to try to find such differentiation with both anti-epithelial membrane antigen and anti-cytokeratin 7 antibodies. Alternatively, anti-CEA antibodies could have been used, but these tend to have a higher level of background staining.

In some cases, Merkel cell carcinoma may also enter into the differential diagnosis. In those cases, anti-CK20 could be added to the panel.

Vignette G

Differential Diagnosis of Dermatofibroma vs Dermatofibrosarcoma Protuberans

A 42-yr-old woman presented to the dermatologist with a multinodular 1.3 cm hyperpigmented growth on her shoulder. She claimed

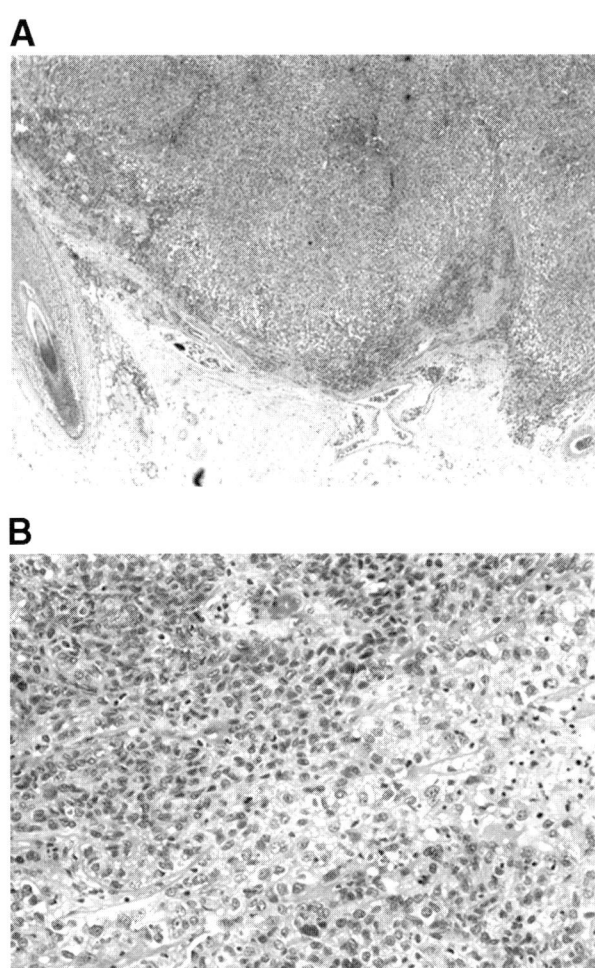

Fig. 11. (A) A tumor comprised of small dark cells coursing throughout the dermis in large nests is present. There is no cleft artifact present surrounding the epithelial islands. **(B)** There are spaces within the epithelial islands. No definitive ductular differentiation is seen.

Table 6
Differential Diagnosis of Basaloid Proliferations

	CAM 5.2	EMA	Cytokeratin 7
Basal cell carcinoma	−	−	−
Eccrine epithelioma	+	+	+

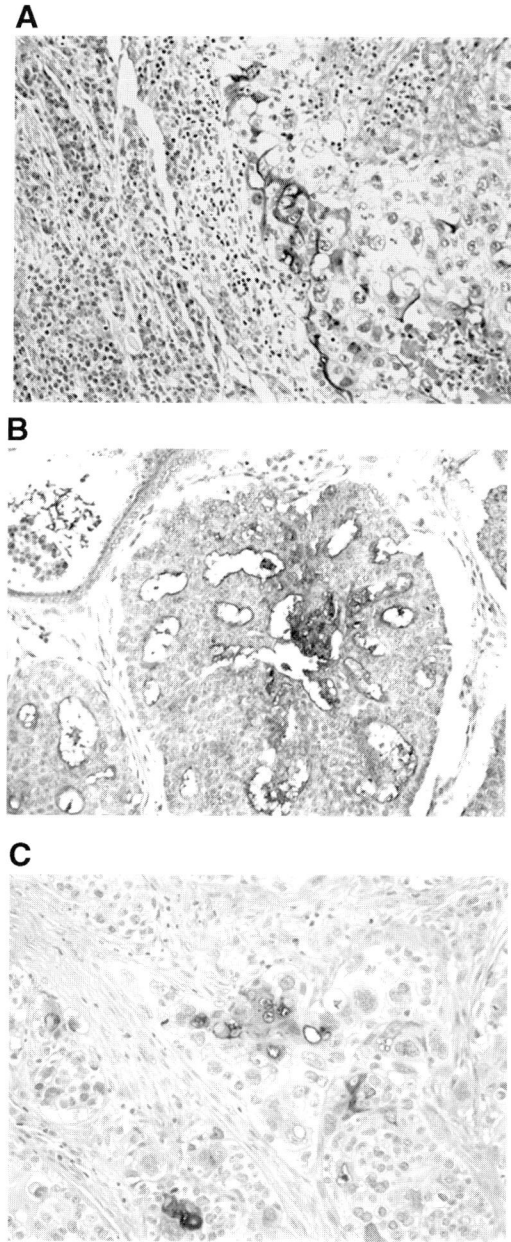

Fig. 12. (A) CAM5.2 strongly labels cells lining the spaces present within the epithelial islands. **(B)** Anti-EMA antibodies are also present in these same ductular lining cells. **(C)** Strong staining with anti-cytokeratin 7 antibodies is present within the cells lining these spaces.

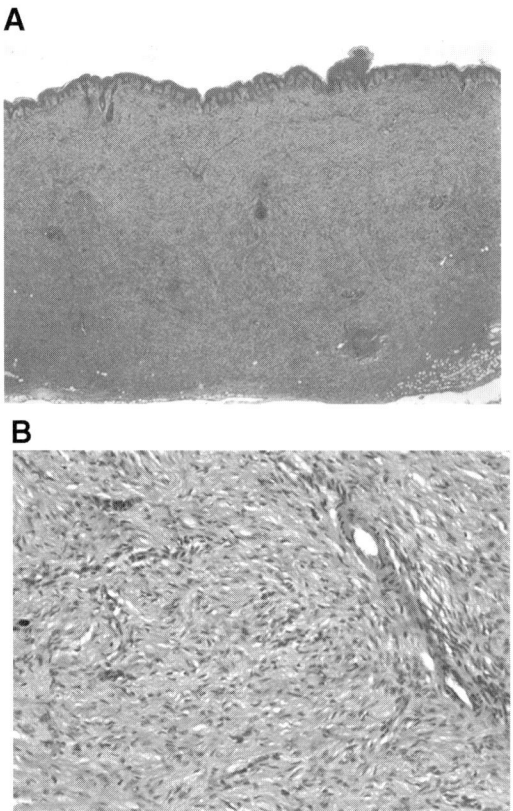

Fig. 13. (A) Within the mid-reticular dermis, there is a cellular proliferation of spindle shaped cells. **(B)** The tumor cells are relatively uniform in appearance and display minimal cytologic atypia. Mitotic activity is very slight.

Table 7
Differential Diagnosis of Bland Spindle Cell Proliferations in the Dermis

	S100	*CD34*	*Factor XIIIa*	*Smooth muscle actin*
Dermatofibrosarcoma protuberans	−	+	−	−
Dermatofibroma	−	−	+	−
Neurofibroma	+	±	−	−
Dermatomyofibroma	−	−	−	+
Leiomyoma	−	−	−	+

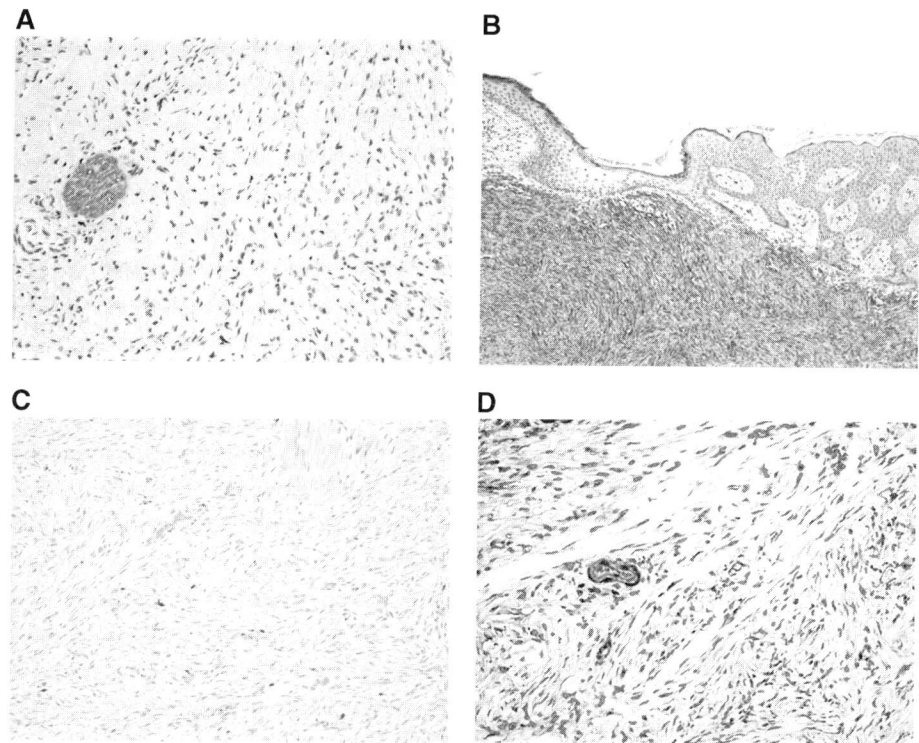

Fig. 14. (A) Anti-S100 protein does not recognize the spindle shaped tumor cells. **(B)** CD34 is strongly expressed by virtually all cells within the tumor. **(C)** Anti-factor XIIIa antibodies demonstrate scattered positive cells, but the majority of the tumor cells fail to express this antigen. **(D)** The tumor cells do not express smooth muscle actin.

that it had been growing slowly over the past 2–3 yr, but could not remember when she first noticed it. The clinical differential diagnosis included a dermatofibroma, dermatofibrosarcoma protuberans, leiomyoma, or other dermal tumor.

Routine histologic sections demonstrated a dermal spindle cell neoplasm, as seen in Fig. 13A,B.

The histologic differential diagnosis included mainly "fibroblast-like" proliferations such as dermatofibroma and dermatofibrosarcoma protuberans. Neural neoplasms seemed less likely. Dermatomyofibroma was also considered in the differential diagnosis. A panel of immunostains shown in Table 7 was developed to solve this diagnostic dilemma.

The results from the immunostaining are seen in Fig. 14A–D. Virtually all dermatofibrosarcoma protuberans stain diffusely with anti-CD34, as is seen in this case. While not usually necessary, in less cellular variants, this stain can be very helpful. In contrast, CD34 staining is rarely present in dermatofibromas. While focal elements of a neurofibroma may express CD34, the focal S100 positivity of the schwann cells will help differentiate this neoplasm. The distinction between a dermatomyofibroma and leiomyoma is more difficult with immunolabeling, but routine histology usually separates these entities. (The newly described anti-caldesmon antibody may prove to be helpful in making this decision.) As both express smooth muscle actin, but not CD34, differentiation from dermatofibrosarcoma protuberans is not a problem.

Vignette H

Differential Diagnosis of Spongiotic Dermatitis in a Child

A 5-wk-old boy was seen in the dermatology clinic with a diffuse erythematous, scaly eruption that was most extensive on his face, neck and scalp. It was not noticed at birth, but appeared within the first week of life and continued to progress. The clinical differential diagnosis included atopic dermatitis, seborrheic dermatitis, and Langerhans cell histiocytosis. The histologic sections prepared from the biopsy specimen are demonstrated in Fig. 15A,B.

The histologic differential diagnosis of a spongiotic process with intraepidermal hematopoietic cells was similar to the clinical differential diagnosis, and included Langerhans cell histocytosis, seborrheic dermatitis, and atopic dermatitis in this patient population. Other entities such as Gianotti-Crosti syndrome and mycosis fungoides were easily eliminated based upon clinical presentation and disease history. A strategic table was developed as is seen in Table 8.

The diagnostic stains are depicted in Fig. 16A,B. It is important to note that Langerhans cells express CD4 and that this antibody cannot be used to differentiate Langerhans cells from intraepidermal T helper lymphocytes. However, they do not express CD3. The key immunostaining result in this case is the strong, diffuse staining of virtually all of the hematopoietic cells with CD1a. It should also be noted that pan T cell markers are expressed by the inflammatory infiltrates in both atopic dermatitis and seborrheic dermatitis. Immunostains are not helpful in making this distinction. (While Langerhans cells may be slightly increased within the epidermis in both diseases, in neither will they represent the dominant hematopoietic cell infiltrate within the epidermis.)

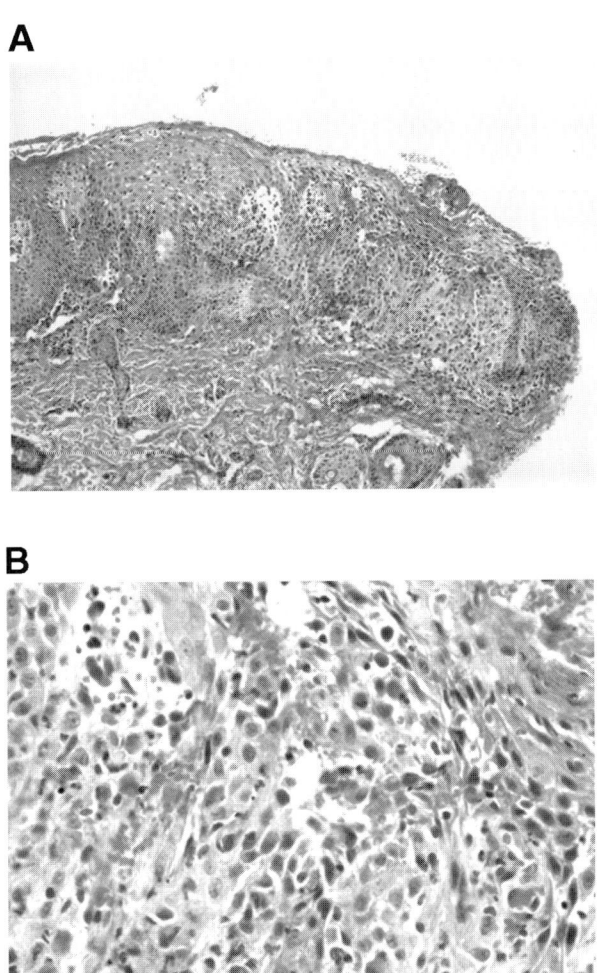

Fig. 15. (A) Histologic sections demonstrate intraepidermal hematopoietic cells with accompanying spongiosis. **(B)** The cells appear slightly enlarged and have a small bit of cytoplasm.

Table 8
Differential Diagnosis of Spongiotic Processes of Childhood

	CD3	CD4	CD1a
Langerhans cell histiocytosis	−	+	+
Atopic dermatitis	+	+	−
Seborrheic dermatitis	+	+	−

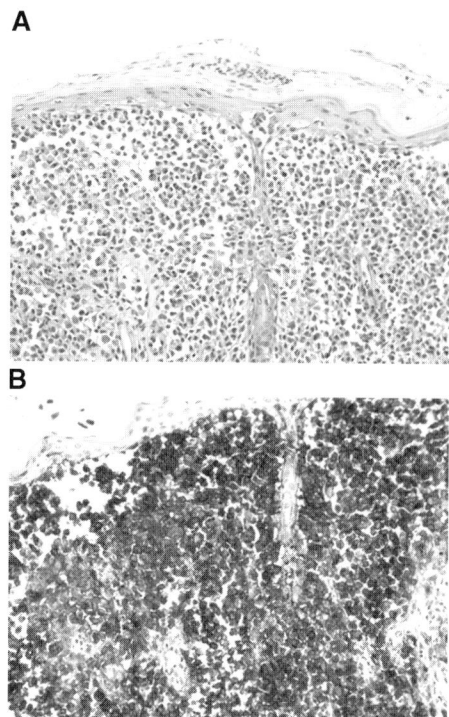

Fig. 16. (A) The intraepidermal cells fail to express CD3. **(B)** There is strong staining with anti-CD1a antibody in the epidermotropic hematopoietic cells.

Vignette I

Differential Diagnosis of an Atypical Lymphoid Infiltrate

A 47-yr-old woman presented to the dermatologist with scattered erythematous papules and nodules on her left arm. Several of them appeared ulcerated. The clinical differential diagnosis included multiple arthropod bites, lymphomatoid papulosis, and pityriasis lichenoides et varioliformis acuta. A biopsy was performed and is shown in Fig. 17A,B.

The histologic differential diagnosis included lymphomatoid papulosis, arthropod bite reaction, pityriasis lichenoides et varioliformis acuta and large cell anaplastic lymphoma. The number of atypical lymphocytes suggested the first diagnosis to be most likely. An antibody panel was developed to confirm this diagnosis.

Figure 18A–C demonstrate the results of the immunolabeling studies. Examination of the constructed panel reveals that all of the

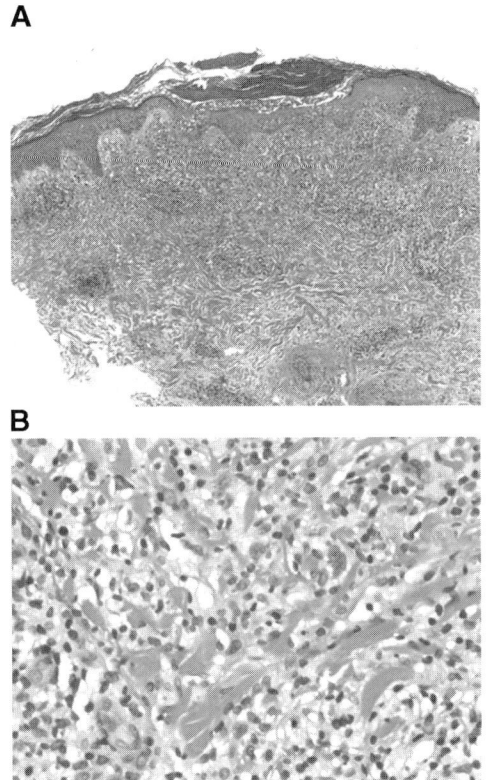

Fig. 17. (A) Histologic sections demonstrate a superficial and deep perivascular infiltrate with focal exocytosis. **(B)** Higher magnification demonstrates focal enlarged, atypical lymphocytes and a mixed inflammatory infiltrate.

Table 9
Differential Diagnosis of Atypical Dermal Lymphocytes

	CD3	CD20	CD7	CD30
Lymphomatoid papulosis	+	–	–	+ (10–20%) of cells
Arthropod bite reaction	+	Rare	+	Rare
Pityriasis lichenoides et varioliformis acuta	+	–	+	Rare
Large cell anaplastic lymphoma	+	– (Extremely rare)	±	+ (>75% of cells)

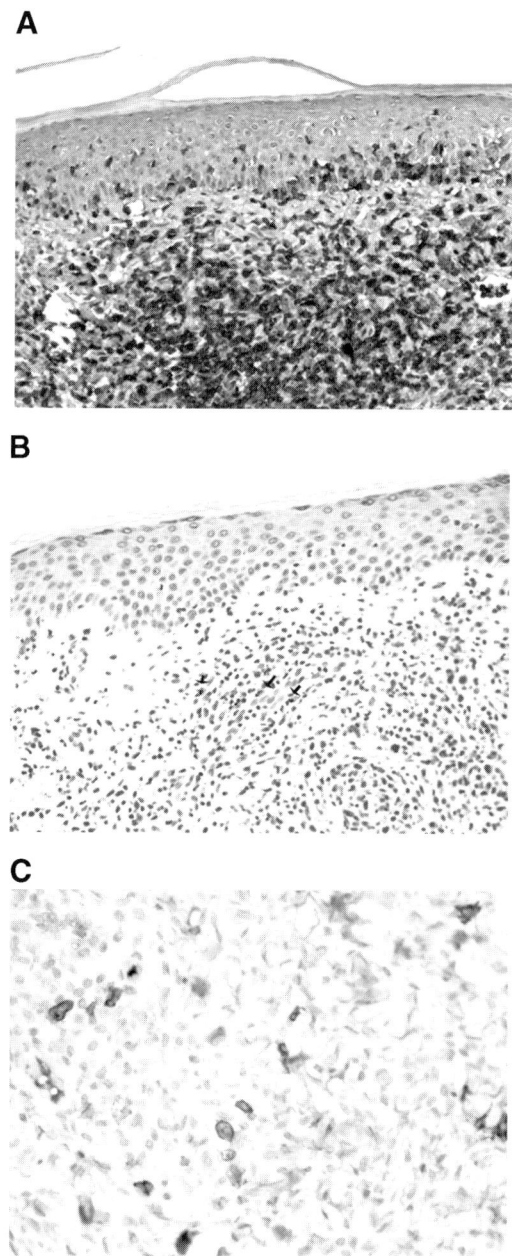

Fig. 18. (A) Anti-CD3 stains virtually all of the inflammatory cells within the dermis. **(B)** Only rare dermal cells express CD20. **(C)** The large, atypical cells within the dermis express CD30, constituting only a minority population of the dermal infiltrate.

processes considered in the differential diagnosis are predominantly T cell processes; however, occasional B cells may be present in an arthropod bite reaction. While CD30 expression is seen in rare cells in arthropod bite reactions and pityriasis lichenoides et varioliformis acuta, such cells rarely exceed 2–5% of infiltrating T lymphocytes. In lymphomatoid papulosis, a significant minority of cells (20–30%), including the atypical cells (especially in type A lymphomatoid papulosis) expresses this antigen. However, in large cell anaplastic lymphoma, by definition more than 75% of the infiltrating T cells express CD30. The major differential diagnoses in this situation are the newly described Type C lymphomatoid papulosis, which can only be distinguished based upon clinical grounds, and a secondary large cell anaplastic lymphoma, which is primarily distinguished by history. (Note that extremely rare cases of large cell anaplastic lymphoma of the skin are comprised of B lymphocytes and not T lymphocytes.)

Vignette J

Differential Diagnosis of an Atypical Dermal Spindle Cell Proliferation

The patient is an 82-yr-old man who presented with an ulcerated nodule on his right ear that had been present for about 6 mo. The clinical differential diagnosis included squamous cell carcinoma, basal cell carcinoma, amelanotic melanoma, and atypical fibroxanthoma. A small shave biopsy was performed yielding the following tissue sections (Fig. 19A,B).

The differential diagnosis of this specimen included spindled squamous cell carcinoma, atypical fibroxanthoma, spindle cell melanoma, and leiomyosarcoma and perhaps poorly differentiated angiosarcoma (though the cells in these neoplasms are not usually quite so spindle-shaped). An immunostaining strategy was established to decipher this differential diagnosis and is portrayed in Table 10.

The immunostaining for this case is shown in Fig. 20A–D. As can be seen, there was staining with CD68 and focally with smooth muscle actin. The CD68 staining is expected in atypical fibroxan-thomas, but can also be seen focally in some cases of melanoma and leiomyosarcoma. The focal staining with smooth muscle actin is not surprising in an atypical fibroxanthoma, but would be unusual in a

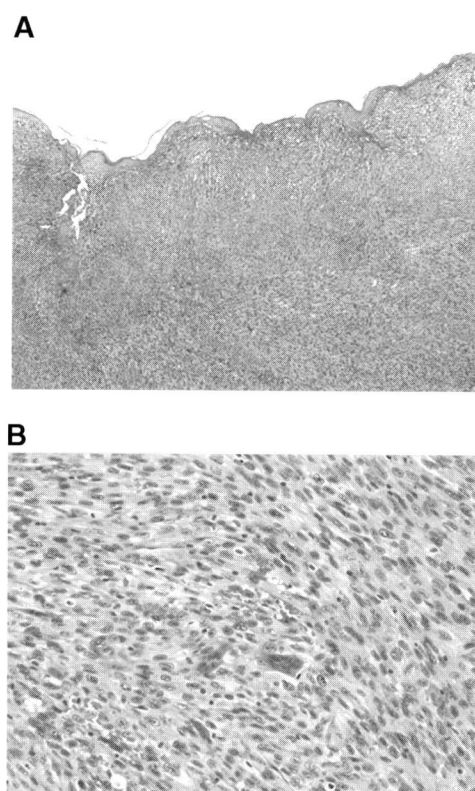

Fig. 19. (A) Low power demonstrates a dermal spindle cell infiltrate with no obvious connection to the overlying epidermis. **(B)** Higher magnification demonstrates marked atypia and scattered multinucleated cells.

Table 10
Differential Diagnosis of Atypical Dermal Spindle Cell Tumor

	S100	CD68	Smooth muscle actin	CD31	Cytokeratin
Atypical fibroxanthoma	−	+	±	−	−
Melanoma	+	±	−	−	−
Squamous cell carcinoma	−	−	−	−	Variable
Leiomyosarcoma	−	±	+	−	−
Angiosarcoma	−	−	−	+	−

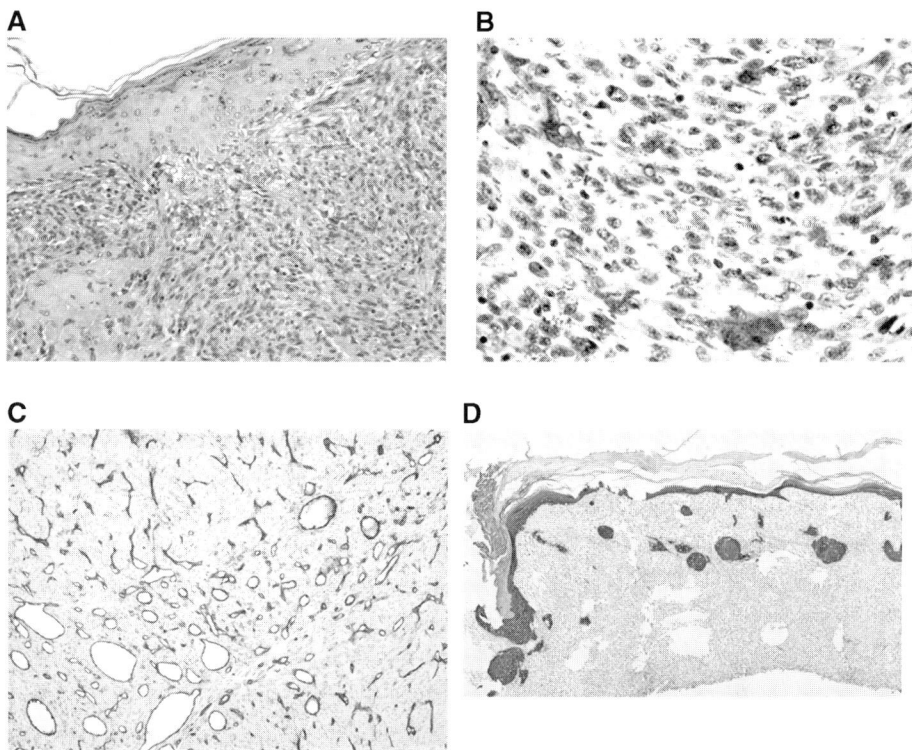

Fig. 20. (A) Anti-S100 fails to stain the population of dermal spindle shaped cells. **(B)** Anti-CD68 antibody identifies only scattered cells in the spindle cell infiltrate. **(C)** CD31 is strongly expressed by dermal endothelial cells, but not by the spindle cells in the tumor. **(D)** Anti-cytokera-tin is strongly expressed by cells in the overlying epidermis, but not in the tumor cells.

melanoma. Leiomyosarcomas are almost always strongly and diffusely positive with this marker and the focal staining seen in this case would be most unusual. The negative S100 is additional evidence against a melanoma. The absence of CD31 staining of the tumor cells, with concomitant strong staining of the dermal blood vessels mitigates against an angiosarcoma. If angiosarcoma were a stronger diagnostic consideration, addition of anti-CD34 antibodies would be helpful in excluding or including endothelial cell differentiation. It is difficult to completely exclude a spindled squamous cell carcinoma. The absence of cytokeratin staining does not exclude this possibility, though the presence of smooth muscle actin and CD68 would be unusual for this diagnosis. (New information suggests that the inclusion of anti-CK5/6 antibodies might be helpful in positively labeling spindle cell squamous cell carcinomas.)

There are several other points worth mentioning. There is little role for antibodies directed against vimentin in this differential diagnosis. With the exception of squamous cell carcinomas, all of the tumors considered would be expected to demonstrate strong cytoplasmic staining. In addition, vimentin can be seen in a significant percentage of spindled squamous cell carcinomas. Thus, a positive result has virtually no discriminatory power. There is also little reason to add MART-1, HMB-45, or any other "melanocyte specific" marker to the panel. Spindle cell melanomas almost always fail to express these antigens. Thus, a negative result would add little information to that attained from the panel as presented.

Vignette K

Differential Diagnosis of Mycosis Fungoides

A 72-yr-old man presented to the dermatology clinic with a known 5-yr history of erythematous patches on his proximal trunk and extremities. The patches initially responded to topical steroids, but more recently persisted even with treatment. The differential diagnosis included contact dermatitis, mycosis fungoides, and a drug eruption. Several punch biopsies were performed and are demonstrated in Fig. 21A,B.

The histologic differential diagnosis included a partially treated spongiotic dermatitis, mycosis fungoides, chronic actinic dermatosis (actinic reticuloid), and perhaps a drug eruption. In order to resolve this differential diagnosis, a panel of immunostains was developed and is presented in Table 11.

Fig. 22A–D demonstrate the immunolabeling results in this case. It is important to note that most inflammatory dermatoses are comprised almost entirely of CD3 positive T cells. CD20 positive B cells represent only a small minority of infiltrating cells. Mycosis fungoides is characterized by a marked predominance of CD4+ T helper lymphocytes. T helper cells are about 10× more frequent than are CD8+ cells in the dermal and epidermal infiltrates in mycosis fungoides, as is seen in this case. In many cases, less than 10% of these cells will express the pan-T cell antigen CD7. This is in contrast to inflammatory processes in which the vast majority of lymphocytes express CD7. Chronic actinic dermatoses are characterized by a predominantly CD8+ cell infiltrate.

A

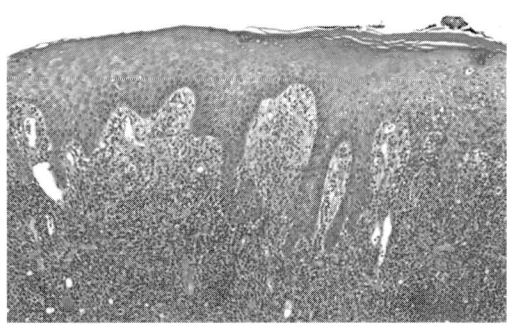

B

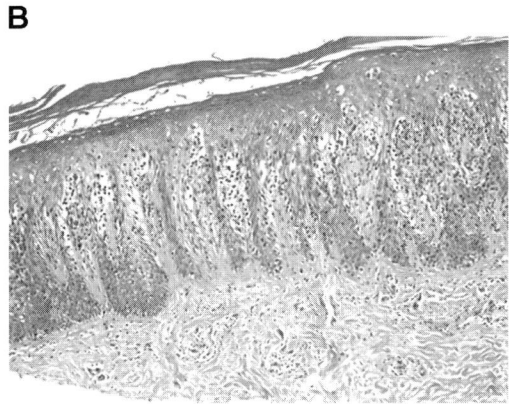

Fig. 21. (A) A band-like infiltrate of lymphocytes is seen along the dermal epidermal junction and there is focal epidermotropism. **(B)** Higher magnification demonstrates dermal fibrosis, epidermotropism and minimal spongiosis.

Table 11
Differential Diagnosis of Mycosis Fungoides

	CD3	CD4	CD8	CD7	CD20
Spongiotic dermatitis	+	+ (Majority)	+ (Minority)	+	−
Chronic actinic dermatosis	+	+ (Minority)	+ (Majority)	+	−
Drug eruption	+	+	+	+	−
Mycosis fungoides	+	+ (Usually >90% of T cells)	+ (Usually <10% of T cells)	−	−

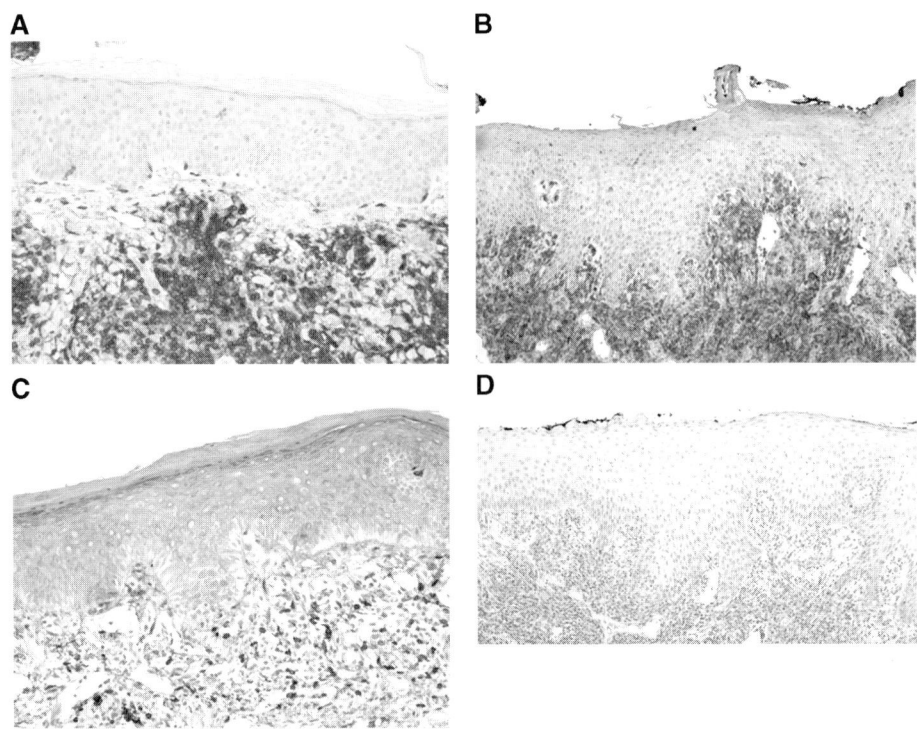

Fig. 22. (A) Anti-CD3 antibodies label virtually all of the lymphocytes in the epidermis and dermis. **(B)** The vast majority of epidermal and dermal lymphocytes expresses CD4. **(C)** A minority population of lymphocytes in this biopsy specimen expresses CD8. **(D)** Only rare cells in the dermis express CD20.

INDEX